Brain and Mind
Made Simple

David Nutt

WATERSIDE PRESS

Brain and Mind Made Simple
David Nutt

ISBN 978-1-914603-00-6 (Paperback)
ISBN 978-1-914603-01-3 (EPUB ebook)
ISBN 978-1-914603-02-0 (PDF ebook)

Main UK distributor Gardners Books, 1 Whittle Drive, Eastbourne, BN23 6QH. Tel: (+44) 01323 521777; sales@gardners.com; www.gardners.com

North American distribution Ingram Book Company, One Ingram Blvd, La Vergne, TN 37086, USA. Tel: (+1) 615 793 5000; inquiry@ingramcontent.com

Cataloguing In-Publication Data A catalogue record for this book can be obtained from the British Library.

Published 2021 by
Waterside Press Ltd
Sherfield Gables
Sherfield on Loddon, Hook
Hampshire RG27 0JG.

Telephone +44(0)1256 882250
Online catalogue WatersidePress.co.uk
Email enquiries@watersidepress.co.uk

All royalties from the sale of this book go to Drug Science.

Table of Contents

Publisher's note

The views and opinions in this book are those of the author and not necessarily shared by the publishers. Whilst every effort has been made to ensure the accuracy of the information contained in the text, readers should draw their own conclusions concerning the possibility of alternative views, accounts, descriptions or explanations.

Acknowledgements

Many people have inspired and supported me in my career as a researcher and psychiatrist. My particular thanks are owed to Professor David Grahame-Smith, Director of the Medical Research Council Clinical Pharmacology Unit in Oxford. He gave me my crucial first break in science by taking me into his unit as a clinical research fellow. And to Dr Richard Green my PhD supervisor who showed great patience as I explored the new world of preclinical neuropsychopharmacology.

I am also particularly grateful to Professor Michael Gelder the head of the Psychiatry Department in Oxford for supporting my transition into clinical research, and the Wellcome Trust for funding me in this.

My grateful thanks are also due to John Lewis, Research Director of Reckitt & Colman for setting up the Bristol University Psychopharmacology Unit that allowed me the independence to develop my own research career.

David Nutt
August 2021

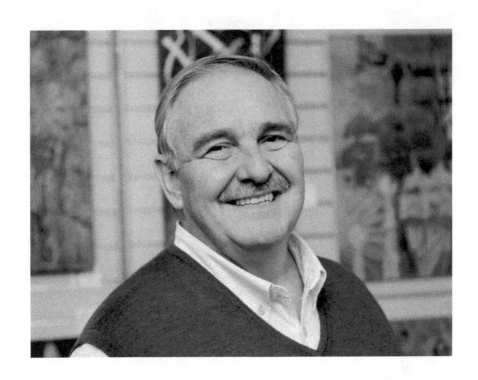

Professor David Nutt

About the author

David Nutt is a Fellow of the Academy of Medical Sciences, founder of Drug Science and Chair of its Scientific Committee.

He is the Edmund J Safra Professor of Neuropsychopharmacology and Head of the Neuropsychopharmacology Unit in the Centre for Academic Psychiatry in the Division of Brain Sciences, Department of Medicine, Hammersmith Hospital, Imperial College London. He is also Visiting Professor at the Open University and Maastricht University in The Netherlands.

His leadership positions include (or have included) the presidencies of the European Brain Council, British Neuroscience Association, British Association of Psychopharmacology and the European College of Neuropsychopharmacology, as well as his time as Chair of the UK's Advisory Council on the Misuse of Drugs.

Most people know David Nutt as the UK's sacked Drug Czar—kicked out for speaking truth to power, i.e. that UK policy on drugs and alcohol was not fit for purpose but driven by politics not science.

But as can be seen above, in a life outside politics, the author is an academic psychiatrist and brain researcher who studies the brain to help understand how it goes awry in mental and neurological illnesses.

A few years ago, before Covid, he started giving public lectures explaining how the brain works and how alterations of the mind can occur as a result of changes in brain function. They were extremely popular—usually over 150 people at each—with lots of questions. So, he decided to write the lectures up in this book for the general public, and anyone else with an interest in the field, especially university students of psychology, medicine and neuroscience.

As well as educating these groups, all royalties from this book will also help support the charity Drug Science that David Nutt set-up after his sacking to continue to promote the cause of bringing scientific evidence to improve drug policy.

His many writings and publications include *Nutt Uncut*, Waterside Press 2020.

This book is dedicated to the memory of my first research supervisors:

David Grahame-Smith, Richard Green and Michael Gelder.

Sadly all now deceased.

And also to Colin Blakemore — an inspiration
since my very first undergraduate days.

Introduction

Most scientists agree that the two last—and arguably greatest—challenges to human comprehension are the origins of the universe and the workings of the human brain. This book is about the nature of the human brain and how modern neuroscience and the study of drugs that alter consciousness have given us new and important insights into how it works.

In the book I describe how the brain is made up of billions of neurons linked together in different systems. I shall explain how the brain is constructed and how the different parts work. This then leads us to understanding the role of the neurotransmitters (chemical messengers that neurons use to communicate with each other). From this we explore the nature of different states of consciousness such as sleep, coma, and mental illnesses.

A bit about myself

It seems that I have always had a fascination with the power of the brain. My mother tells me that when aged ten I was interviewed by a local newspaper about some calculations I had done on the volume of rain that fell each year on our school playground (as we lived in the West of England that was a lot). Apparently, I told them my ambition was to be a scientist and understand how the brain works. I have been fortunate in knowing what I wanted to do from an early age and being allowed to pursue this ambition. I hope I have added to our knowledge and understanding of brain function, particularly in relation to pharmacological research and the treatment of psychiatric disorders.

A major influence in encouraging me to pursue this research path came from a school visit of the Sixth Form Science Club to the lab of Professor William Grey Walter at the Burden Neurological Institute in my home city of Bristol. Grey Walter was one the pioneers of human neuroscience. He developed the early technology for measuring EEG (brain waves) and the changes provoked by sensory input (evoked potentials), even those originating in the brain in anticipation of action. He also built the first self-fuelling robot that would locate a power socket to recharge itself when its battery was running low. His 1950s book *The Living Brain* (see *Selected Bibliography*) opened my mind to the opportunities and needs for clinical brain research.

It encouraged me into medicine rather than just pure neuroscience research despite my having met at Cambridge University the doyen of UK neuroscience, the other Huxley brother Andrew. He won the Nobel Prize in medicine and physiology in 1963, along with one of my Cambridge teachers Alan Hodgkin, for describing the mathematics of the nerve action potential and then went on to revolutionise our understanding of how muscles contract.

Overall, the Huxley brothers can be seen as the two poles of neuroscience. At one end was Andrew with the maths and physics of how neurons work and at the other Aldous,[1] who explained how the collection of billions of neurons we call the brain produce consciousness and personal meaning.

For the next 40 years I developed my career as a student, doctor, psychiatrist, researcher and academic. I will describe in more detail in the book how, as a doctor, I have seen patients experience days of profound hallucinations and delusions under the influence of toxic doses of older antidepressants taken in attempted suicides. I have seen people with brain tumours develop completely different personalities—to the horror of their families, though with no insight themselves. I have seen people in delirium attack staff trying to help them, then have no recollection of their behaviour when the infection has subsided. I have myself been fought off by a diabetic man with extreme life-threatening hypoglycaemia who had no insight that without my intervention he would likely die. With his wife's help I held him down, injected him intravenously with glucose, and watched him return to normality in seconds, with no recollection of his violent opposition just a minute before.

In the clinic I have watched a man with temporal lobe epilepsy have a fit in front of me during which he wandered around the room rubbing his nose and then came out of it and asked why we had changed our seats.

As a clinical psychopharmacologist (someone who studies the effects of drugs on the brain) my research involves the use of drugs to explore how the human

---

1.   The author of *Brave New World* and *The Doors of Perception* (see *Selected Bibliography*).

mind and brain work and how they might go wrong in psychiatric disorders. I have given (often to myself as well as other volunteers) a range of drugs that had profound effects on the brain and body. I have seen some people release huge secret emotional tensions under the influence of benzodiazepines whereas others just become sleepy and confused.

As a psychiatrist I have interviewed people with grandiose feelings and beliefs under the influence of stimulants such as cocaine yet also seen other people paranoid and aggressive from taking the same drug. I have watched patients acting through severe hallucinations during the delirium induced by alcohol or benzodiazepine withdrawal or tricyclic antidepressant overdose. I have observed patients with anxiety getting worse over the first few days of treatment with antidepressants that then within a few more weeks make them dramatically better.

In studies on addiction, I have given heroin addicts an intravenous (IV) dose of heroin in the lab and observed them stop breathing for 20 seconds or more, completely unaware of this and unconcerned. When we remind them to start breathing again, they do so without any sense of discomfort at having stopped. In contrast I have seen patients with panic attacks be unable to hold their breath for even a few seconds without a terrible fear that they were suffocating. Yet a few weeks later, on effective treatment, they could do the test with ease. The range of abilities of the brain is awe-inspiring and immense. In this book I try to make sense of this from a neurobiological perspective.

PART 1

HOW THE BRAIN WORKS

CHAPTER 1

The Origins of Our Brains — Ions, Membranes and Pumps

As I said in my *Introduction*, most scientists agree that the two last—and greatest—challenges to human comprehension are the origins of the universe and the workings of the human brain. The human brain is generally accepted as the most complex single entity in existence. But we, the human species, are massively more powerful and complex. When we put all our brain power together, working with the knowledge accumulated by the billions of human brains that have ever existed, and with their legacies in literature and science, humankind has truly remarkable intellectual capacity. We can generate evidence for theories that explain the origins of matter and of life, develop machines and communications systems that can escape our solar system and penetrate the outer edges of our universe, and invent weapons that could destroy the world, including ourselves. We can even change our genetic material so now can (if we wanted to) direct our own evolution.

All this comes because we have a special brain that not only has remarkable capacities, particularly for language, but also has evolved to make us share knowledge and interests and work together in powerful social organizations we call society. So how did humankind get to this pre-eminent position in the universe? How did our human brain evolve?

The beginnings of life are thought to be due to the emergence, several billions of years ago, of chemical molecules such as amino-acids, fats and sugars in some sort of chemical solution. These chemicals were probably derived from reactions promoted by electricity from lightning and heat from volcanic eruptions, though some think they arrived from other more evolved planets via asteroids. Whatever their origin, through further chemical reactions these first simple molecules gradually fused and grew into more complex and larger ones. These eventually developed the remarkable capacity for replication and self-assembly into larger molecules particularly proteins and DNA/RNA that began life as we know it today because of their ability to self-replicate and so produce identical copies of themselves for evermore. Ribonucleic acid (RNA) is an important biological macromolecule that is present in all biological cells. It is principally involved in the synthesis of proteins, carrying the messenger instructions from DNA, which itself contains the genetic instructions required for the development and maintenance of life.

The DNA/RNA set of large molecules were unarguably the critical phase in the evolution of life. These molecules have several remarkable properties. Foremost is the ability to reproduce faithful copies of themselves, so transferring their structure from generation to generation. The best example of this is DNA but both RNA and proteins can do the same to a lesser extent. The second truly remarkable development was the evolution of DNA to code for RNA and then RNA to code for proteins. Proteins are the core ingredients of life as they make up the enzymes that control all metabolic processes as well as the pumps and other cell surface elements such as receptors that we shall see later are the necessary components of communication. The language of DNA is the most remarkable development as through just four 'letters' it gives an enormous variety of different RNA and thus protein combinations.

Perhaps even more remarkably, an as yet unexplained transition occurred in which individual molecules came together in a tiny living bubble that we now call a cell. These contain DNA so were able to self-replicate and thus life as we know it emerged (all living things are collections of individual cells). These tiny bubbles of life had an outer cell membrane of lipid (fat) plus protein combinations that kept inside it the inner chemical workings of the cell. These then provided energy and the apparatus necessary for cell replication which was some early variant of DNA. These original single cells were the precursors of the bacteria and amoebae we have today. Growth and mutations of DNA and RNA continued over billions of years and resulted the development of new proteins with new properties and so evolution continued.

The next major advance in terms of our story of the nervous system was the emergence of a new kind of protein, one that spanned the cell membrane. These proteins developed the ability to pump certain electrically charged atoms (ions) into or out of the cell and are therefore called 'ion pumps' or 'ion channels.' Their pumping activity allowed the creation of concentrations and gradients of ions between the inside and the outside of the cell membrane. These pumps and ion gradients are still vital to the function of all cells today and they are the foundation of the core processes by which nerve cells work.

In essence cells pump sodium and calcium ions out of the cell and concentrate potassium inside them. Biological fluids found outside the cell, including our blood, mirror the salt (sodium chloride) solution found in the sea (which makes sense as that's where the first cells lived). This high sodium concentration is not conducive to most biological processes. We often use strong salt solutions as disinfectants or to preserve food, e.g. salted-cod, as it stops bacteria growing. Keeping salt out of cells via these pumps is therefore vital for the enzymes and other processes inside the cell to work properly.

Once there is a sufficient concentration difference of sodium between the inside and outside of the cell then this results in an electrical potential across the cell membrane (called the membrane potential) that is found in all living cells. As we shall discover later, this membrane potential is harnessed to make other activities in the cell happen.

In a few more billion years these single cells developed the ability to come together as larger groups as we see in slime moulds and coral today. Then from these larger clusters, probably from mutations within single cells, some specialisation of cell functions developed. A good example is in the simple animal called hydra. These have wavy tentacle-like extensions (flagellae) that project out into the sea from their central cylindrical core or 'mouth.' These flagellae can catch food and then pull it into the 'mouth.' The flagellae move if the ion balance in their cells is altered. Food touching the flagellae, or chemicals from creatures in the vicinity, trigger changes in the membrane pumps so that sodium and calcium ions enter the cell. The calcium ions then activate proteins, precursors of those found in our present-day muscles, that then contract and move the flagellae to catch the food and bring it into the mouth.

Subsequently, some cells started specialising in managing ion movements and they also began to elongate, becoming precursors of those that we now call nerve cells or neurons. These are the specialised cells from which our brains and nervous systems are made up and they have the special property of conducting electricity along their length—the nerve impulse or action potential. This allows them to transmit information long distances like in a telegraph wire (see *Figure 1*).

Action potentials are electrical currents that run the length of the neuron and are produced by the opening of sodium channels (a process we call depolarisation) in the neuronal membrane so that electrical current flows into the neuron and this then opens more channels, so the current is perpetuated along the length of the nerve. The longest neurons in humans run from the spinal cord to the tip of the toes—and are even longer in bigger animals but can conduct an action potential along their total length in a few thousandths of a second.

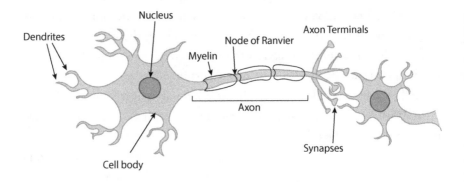

Figure 1: A neuron connecting to another neuron

Further specialisation then developed with some neurons evolving to be dedicated to receiving information from the outside world and others to controlling movements; these are the precursors of the present-day sensory and motor systems in our central nervous system (CNS).

The evolution of the nervous system demonstrates that the first neuronal activity developed to enable movement to catch food and so grow and reproduce. All the super-complexity of the brain that has evolved since then is just a sophisticated elaboration of this original primitive role; nerves allow animals to move so make more efficient their search for food! Because plants make their own food they don't need to move so have no or very rudimentary (e.g. those that close the leaves of a venous fly trap) nervous systems at best.

One important other aspect of neuronal activity is that it never stops — until we die. This ceaseless activity of neurons is due to ions leaking into neurons and causing them to keep firing. It is vital to allow the fundamental unconscious processes, especially breathing and heart beating, to continue even when we are asleep or in a coma. But this ceaseless activity also happens in many other neurons and this is responsible for the perpetual ongoing activity of higher brain functions such as movement, exploration and ultimately in the human brain the seeking of novel experiences and knowledge and understanding. These occur just as much in sleep as when we are awake and explain dreams and the common experience that we can go to bed with a problem in our mind and wake up with a solution.

As we shall discover later, quite a lot of brain function then becomes involved in controlling and regulating this ceaseless neuronal firing, and if the correct balance of activity and regulation is not achieved or maintained then disorders of behaviour and thinking can emerge.

Communicating with chemicals

The other major innovation that underpins current brain function is that of chemical neurotransmission. Primitive neurons as well as having powerful ion fluxes also developed a means of communicating between each other by releasing chemicals that could diffuse across the space between cells (which in the nervous system is called the 'synapse': see *Figures 1* and *5*) to activate or inhibit the other neurons they engage with.

These chemicals we now call neurotransmitters. Over time neurons developed means to store them so there were plenty ready for use when the neuron needed to release them. Neurotransmitters are concentrated in small spherical sacs (called 'vesicles') which are congregated at the end of the neuron (see *Figure 2*). When the neuronal action potential reaches the terminal processes of the axon these vesicles fuse with the neuronal cell membrane. They then open inside-out and so release their neurotransmitter contents into the synapse. Neurotransmitters act on receptors on the downstream neuron and so information is passed around the CNS.

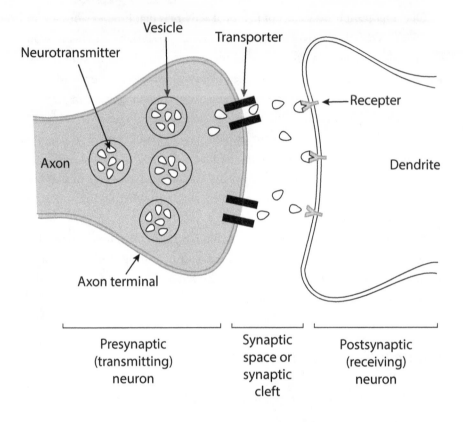

Figure 2: A synapse

If the neurotransmitter stimulates the next neuron, we call this excitation, and if it restrains the activity of the receiving neuron, we call it inhibition. Excitation can be passed on from neuron to neuron in series, travelling from neuron to neuron throughout the organism's CNS. This process of transferring information between neurons by neurotransmitters is still the key to most human brain functions. All that has changed in the past billion years is that upwards of 80 different chemicals have become adopted as neurotransmitters, most stored in its own special vesicles. As we shall see later some of these are excitatory and others inhibitory, so allowing more balanced and integrated responding.

This linking-up of activity of chains of neurons provided a quantum leap in the ability of an organism to coordinate its responses to capture food or to avoid threat. The earliest nervous systems were designed to detect food, direct movement towards it, and then catch it. Subsequently some neurons developed the ability to detect either pressure from creatures bumping into the organism, or chemicals released by them, and so the hydra could respond to the presence of possible prey by moving their flagellae to capture it. These detecting neurons eventually developed into sense-specific organs such as our skin touch sensors and our eyes and ears, so providing much more sophisticated multimodal inputs about the environment. Such sensory inputs improve the organism's responses to vital needs, e.g. food, drink, reproductive mating, and urgent escape from threats.

To improve and optimise the organism's responses in search of food and escape from threats more sophisticated arrangements of neurons developed. This came first in the shape of localised collections of neurons called ganglia — the early precursors of our brains. These neuronal clusters worked together to analyse and integrate the inputs of multiple neurons before preparing outputs.

Often different neurotransmitters were used to make the computation of inputs and outputs. Also, neurons developed in size and complexity. They began to develop multiple branches that allowed them to communicate with many more neurons. Some of these specialised branching processes are called dendrites. These sprout from one end of neurons to allow them to collect information from many thousands of other neurons. At the other end of their cell body neurons developed a single output process called an axon that in some cases can extend many centimetres though the brain or spinal cord to communicate with distant neurons (*Figure 1*).

The dendrites collect information from other neurons and then process it to a decision point when the neuron then either fires off action potentials or not. At the simplest level this can be just a summation of excitatory and inhibitory inputs with the largest total winning. However, we now know that in some cases more complex computation is performed in different parts of the dendritic tree. Also, some inhibitory neurons specifically target the output axons so giving a further level of control of excitatory outputs.

The human brain has grown to be much larger than those of related primates. It has roughly 200 billion neurons and a similar number of supporting cells, called 'glia.' Each neuron has on average a thousand connections with other neurons so the total number of synapses is around 10^{15}. This prodigious number of connections explains its enormous analytical and processing power.

Remarkably the efficiency of the brain in terms of energy use per computation is at least ten times more than that of the best modern computers. This remarkable efficiency of the human brain is why the European Commission for Information Technology has funded the Human Brain Project to the tune of hundreds of millions of euros. The ambition of this megaproject is to decode the way the brain computes and then, from this insight, develop new more powerful and energy-efficient computers and software.

CHAPTER 2

Neurotransmitters and their Receptors — The Locks and Keys of Brain Function

O ne of the most remarkable aspects of the evolution of our nervous system has been the large number of different neurotransmitters that have developed; it is estimated that over 80 different sorts exist in the human brain. Some, e.g. serotonin and noradrenaline, have become household names because of their association with depression and stress reactions respectively. Others, e.g. tachykinins and dynorphins are hardly known at all outside the scientific world despite their having critical roles in pain and mood.

We still are not sure exactly why so many neurotransmitters exist, or even if we have identified all of them! It seems likely there may be a degree of 'belts and braces' in play here, with several different neurotransmitters serving similar, parallel functions. For instance, at least eight different neurotransmitters are known to be involved in maintaining wakefulness, probably because this is so essential for the survival of the organism that it can't risk one neurotransmitter failing and having no back up! What appears to have occurred is that during evolution different chemicals involved initially in metabolic (biochemical) processes inside the cell became 'captured' and turned into neurotransmitters. The most beautiful example is that of gamma aminobutyric acid (GABA) and glutamate described in the next section.

Receptors are specialised small regions of proteins that are embedded in the cell-membrane (see *Figure 3*). Parts of these proteins extrude outside the cell membrane and into the extracellular space into which the neurotransmitters are released, just like the pumps do (*Chapter 1*). In fact, many receptors evolved from these pump proteins. When the neurotransmitter hits the receptor, this acts like a key in a lock; when the two fit together the neurotransmitter is said to bind to the receptor. This binding process changes the conformation of the receptor protein so that the part of it inside the neuron can now change metabolic functions in the neuron. These changes can either excite (turn on) or inhibit (turn off) the neuron on which the receptor is based.

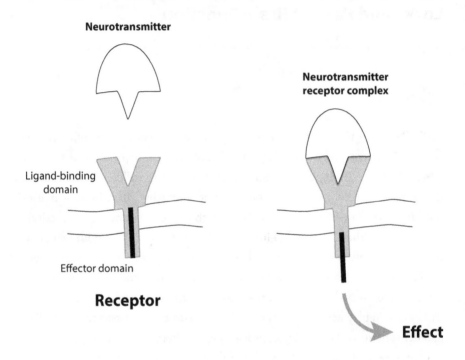

Figure 3: How receptors interact with neurotransmitters

A remarkable recent discovery is that many neurotransmitter receptors are derived from a single adaptable protein that is one of the keys to life on earth—bacterial rhodopsin. This is the protein that in bacteria converts sunlight into energy.

Until rhodopsin evolved all bacteria derived energy from heat or chemical sources. Now the ones with this new protein could use the near limitless energy from the sun to grow and reproduce—just like plants do today when they use chlorophyll to convert sunlight to intracellular energy. Bacterial rhodopsin was the first way light was converted into life. This increase in energy led to a massive increase in the growth of bacteria that then evolved into all the life we have on earth today. If light was not exactly the beginning of life as the *Bible* says, it soon became one of the key factors in developing the many life forms on earth leading to plant growth through chlorophyll and animal brain function through neurotransmission via rhodopsin-derived receptors.

Like all proteins bacterial rhodopsin continued to mutate and as it did variants sensitive to chemicals rather than light evolved. These chemicals became neurotransmitters and the rhodopsin protein their receptors. A whole series of these different receptors developed, and these became, alongside pumps, the other key elements in neuronal function.

The majority of different types of receptors in the nervous system are derived from this bacterial protein, with the others mostly being derived from mutations of pumps. Those receptors related to pumps are called ionotropic receptors because when the neurotransmitter key opens the receptor lock ions flow in or out of the neuron changing the electrical potential across it to make it more or less likely to fire off action potentials.

The other group of receptors that evolved from rhodopsin are called metabotropic receptors (often called G-protein receptors or GPCRs) because the effects they produce are mediated by altering enzyme activity (i.e. metabolism) inside neurons. The most obvious differences between these two sorts of receptors are in their speed of action. Ionotropic receptors, because they produce ion fluxes across the neuronal cell membrane result in very rapid responses in neurons, of the order of milliseconds. Metabotropic receptors produce slower and often more enduring effects over seconds to hours.

When a neurotransmitter has bound to its receptor it soon dissociates from it and returns back into the synaptic cleft. Then three things can happen, it can bind to the receptor again or it can be taken back into the neuron from which it was released and either broken down (metabolised) or put back into the vesicles for future use. Neurons have developed specialised pumps that can suck back neurotransmitters from the synaptic cleft and these are called reuptake pumps or transporters: see *Figure 1*.

In the same way that metabotropic receptors developed from bacterial rhodopsin, so these reuptake pumps developed from the pumps that bacteria use to protect them from antibiotic toxicity—they are the means by which bacteria develop antibiotic resistance. Of course, these were present millions of years before humans invented antibiotics because bacteria have for billions of years been in a life and death struggle with other sorts of bugs and fungi. These secrete toxins to kill off competitors and these toxins work after they enter the bacteria to damage their metabolism and then kill them (just like modern antibiotics). To stay alive bacteria developed pumps that can extrude these toxins.

At some stage in evolution higher animals adopted these pumps and reversed them so that they pump neurotransmitters into neurons rather than out of them. We know this because the genes coding for neurotransmitter reuptake pumps are of the same family as those that code for the bacteria drug-resistance pumps.

GABA and glutamate — The yin and yang of brain activity

These are two amino-acids that are necessary partners in a key metabolic cycle in the cell, with glutamate being turned into gamma aminobutyric acid (GABA) by an enzyme called glutamic acid decarboxylase (GAD). At some point in evolution one or other of these common and vital cellular chemicals became utilised as a neurotransmitter in addition to it continuing to have a metabolic function. The other was also then made into a neurotransmitter with exactly the opposite actions. Thus, organisms always had a good supply of each to hand, for the amounts needed for neurotransmission are tiny compared with those in the metabolic pool.

In humans and all other mammals, glutamate is the main excitatory neurotransmitter (*Figure 4*). When it is released from one neuron it activates (excites) its target neurons so making them in turn fire off action potentials. As explained above therefore GABA then came to be used to provide the opposite effect—inhibition. In the brain GABA is the main inhibitory neurotransmitter so when released it stops other neurons firing. The human brain is organized so that—whenever glutamate is released to excite the brain—GABA is also released to inhibit the same neurons and so prevent over excitation.

Strangely, in invertebrates and crustaceans, e.g. insects and lobsters, the roles of these two neurotransmitters are reversed—glutamate is inhibitory and GABA is excitatory. This is an important message that tells us the function of a neurotransmitter cannot be simply defined by its chemistry or structure. Neurotransmitter actions depend totally on the effect produced by the receptors that the neurotransmitters act on. Later we shall see that serotonin acts on up to 15 different subtypes of serotonin receptor some of which are excitatory and some inhibitory depending on what other proteins in the neuron the receptor influences.

In the mammalian brain getting this yin-yang balance between excitation (glutamate) and inhibition (GABA) is vital. Too much excitatory activity can lead to neurons dying and too little to the organism being sedated or even asleep. Excess glutamate activity is a major problem after a stroke when the vast metabolic pool of glutamate is released from dying neurons when they can't keep the pumps working to keep it in the vesicles. This wave of glutamate then kills other neurons which then release their glutamate and so on. The size of the stroke expands over a period of several days as glutamate gradually kills more and more neurons in the brain. But too much inhibition is also a problem as can be seen when people die of over-sedation as a result of taking GABA-mimicking drugs such as alcohol and gamma hydroxybutyrate (GHB). Excess inhibition stops the breathing centre.

Optimal brain function therefore depends on the delicate balance between glutamate excitation and GABA inhibition being perfectly maintained. When one is released the release of the other quickly follows. This is so vital a balancing act that almost all glutamate-releasing neurons also activate many GABA-releasing ones to minimise the risk of over-excitation and neuronal death — see *Figure 4*.

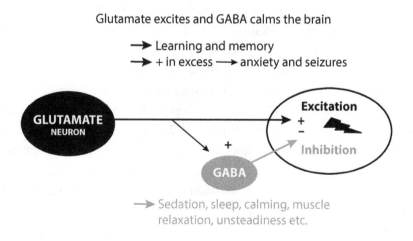

Figure 4: Glutamate and GABA — The on and off of neuron activity

Because they are the prototypical neurotransmitters that have been used in this role for billions of years, both glutamate and GABA have developed relationships with a number of different ionotropic and metabotropic receptors. Glutamate acts on three different ionotropic receptors (AMPA, NMDA, kainate) and at least six metabotropic ones. GABA has just one inotropic one (the GABA-A receptor) and one metabotropic one (the GABA-B receptor). But there are many subtypes of the GABA-A receptor with different brain locations that give a great deal more subtlety to the actions of GABA.

One of the ionotropic receptors glutamate acts on is called the AMPA receptor (if you really want to know what this stands for its α-amino-3-hydroxy-5-methyl-4-isoxazolepropionic acid — don't say you weren't warned!). AMPA receptor stimulation by glutamate opens sodium channels and so produces a rapid excitation of the neurons the receptors are located on. In contrast when the NMDA receptor is stimulated it opens a calcium channel which as well as powerfully exciting the neuron has longer lasting effects described below.

Because the effects of calcium influx into the neuron are so powerful the NMDA receptor is blocked most of the time by the metal ion magnesium. This magnesium block means that the NMDA receptor can only open its calcium channel when neurons are strongly depolarised. This usually occurs when a lot of AMPA receptors are activated at once to massively depolarise the neuron and so force the magnesium off the NMDA receptor. Stimulation of the NMDA receptor by glutamate now opens its calcium channel and allows this ion to flood into the neuron. Calcium entry leads to the laying down of memories because calcium activates enzymes in the neuron that produce long-lasting changes in neuronal connections (so called synaptic plasticity). However excessive calcium influx will damage and eventually kill neurons.

Drugs that block NMDA receptors such as alcohol and ketamine can cause profound amnesia through preventing NMDA receptor activation. They can also dampen the brain to a point where consciousness is lost which is why they can be used as anaesthetics. Though alcohol is rarely used for this purpose today it was until the middle of the 1800s, when nitrous oxide came along, the only anaesthetic for any kind of surgery.

The magnesium block of the NMDA receptor is of huge clinical relevance because magnesium is a vital element in food and if people are magnesium deficient then their brains are more excitable, and they become liable to having seizures (fits). Magnesium deficiency is common in alcohol addiction and explains the hyper-excitable state seen in alcohol withdrawal. It also can occur in the pre-eclampsia of pregnancy which often results in seizures. In both these states, before we had modern anti-convulsant medications, intravenous infusions of magnesium salts were used and often saved lives, and they are still used for these medical emergencies in some low-income countries today.

GABA acting on the GABA-A type of receptor has exactly the opposite effect of glutamate—it is inhibitory. The mechanism is that when the GABA neurotransmitter binds to this receptor it opens a channel that allows the influx of chloride and bicarbonate ions into the neuron. These are negatively (-ve) charged ions so as their concentration increases in the neuron the inside of the cell become more negatively charged. The more of the negative charge there is inside a neuron the harder it is for it to be depolarised (activated), i.e. the more inhibited it is. GABA therefore calms the brain by inhibition of neurons (making them less likely to fire) whereas glutamate has the opposite action, making them more excitable (more likely to fire)—the yin-yang process in action again.

Drugs that enhance the actions of GABA such as benzodiazepines (e.g. Valium) are anxiolytic and conversely drugs that reduce the effects of GABA cause anxiety. We know this because some compounds with these properties have been made for other purposes such as memory enhancers and have demonstrated these adverse effects (and so are no longer in development!). The opposite is true for glutamate—drugs that block glutamate receptors, e.g. ketamine can reduce anxiety and experimental drugs that increase glutamate can cause anxiety.

Alcohol has a 'double whammy' effect on this system. At low doses—1–2 units (15–10gms) that produce a blood alcohol level of 40–100 mg/dL (mg%) it enhances the actions of GABA at the GABA-A receptor to reduce anxiety. This explains why alcohol is so popular at parties where many of us use it to overcome the natural social anxiety about talking to strangers. Alcohol dissolves this social anxiety in the same way as it calms the anxiety of air-passengers who dislike flying, which is why the first thing that happens on aeroplanes once the seat belt sign is switched-off is that drinks are served. But at higher concentrations (blood alcohol >150 mg%) alcohol begins to block the NMDA receptor leading to memory block which we colloquially call 'blackouts.' When alcohol levels get above about 400mg% (as would occur after drinking a litre of vodka) then these two effects of alcohol—the increase in GABA inhibition and the block of glutamate—can combine to produce a lethal level of sedation and respiratory depression such as that which is reported to have killed the popular 27-year-old UK singer Amy Winehouse.

Glutamate blockers (also called antagonists) and GABA activators (also called agonists) have important medical uses. Many anaesthetics and anti-epilepsy drugs act to either block glutamate either directly at glutamate receptors (e.g. ketamine, perampanel) or indirectly (isoflurane, halothane, lamotrigine) or increase GABA (e.g. benzodiazepines, propofol, barbiturates). Benzodiazepines also are powerful muscle relaxants and sleep-inducers via the same mechanisms.

These pharmacological insights have raised the question to what extent could alterations in these receptors and neurotransmitters underlie the brain disorders that the drugs acting on them treat? Modern neuroscientific techniques such as PET brain imaging (see *Chapter 9*) have shown us that patients with severe anxiety such as panic disorder have a relative deficiency of GABA receptors in the brain regions controlling the brain's emotional and physiological responses to fear. Thus, they can't adequately suppress normal fearful responses. In certain forms of epilepsy where there is a localised brain site from which the seizures originate (so called 'focal epilepsy') a deficit in GABA inhibition can also be seen. This form of PET imaging of GABA receptors is now used in specialised centres that conduct epilepsy surgery to define the areas of the brain that can be removed to stop them producing seizures.

In both these conditions a deficit of GABA receptors is believed to lead to reduced inhibition and so a hyper-excitatory state emerges that is expressed as fear or epilepsy depending on where in the brain the changes occur. This theory is now testable in mice where it is possible to produce genetic mutations that result in reduced GABA receptor expression in the brain and, as predicted, these mice are more anxious. In some patients with epilepsy a genetic variation in ion channel function can lead to excessive glutamate excitatory neuronal activity and thus to seizures. These forms of epilepsy too can be replicated in mice by making the same mutations of the ion channel genes and so these mutant mice can be used to screen drugs in the search for new treatments.

There is not time or space to cover all the 80 or so known neurotransmitters and their receptors, but in the rest of this chapter I highlight some that are particularly relevant to the rest of this book and which have gained some interest in popular consciousness.

Serotonin — The many-faceted neurotransmitter

Serotonin (also known as 5-hydroxytryptamine or 5-HT) is a neurotransmitter that is widely known to the public in relation to the treatment of depression. In my psychiatry clinic it was not uncommon for patients with depression to ask if they could have something to treat their self-diagnosed 'serotonin deficiency.' The reality is that still we do not know which cases of depression are directly related to a deficit in serotonin though we have evidence that some are.

What is very clear is that drugs that enhance the effects of serotonin in the synaptic cleft, particularly those that block its reuptake — the so-called selective serotonin reuptake inhibitors or SSRIs (e.g. Prosac, Seroxat, Cipralex) — are effective medicines for depression (antidepressants). These have a particularly powerful therapeutic ability to prevent people having future recurrences (relapses) of their depression.

We also know that deficits in some serotonin receptors, particularly the 5-HT1A receptor are linked to having a familial vulnerability to being depressed or having anxiety states. Low levels of this particular serotonin receptor also contribute to having a family propensity to depression. However, the large number of serotonin receptors — there are at least 15 of them — and the fact that some are inhibitory and others excitatory means that one cannot simply speak of an 'action' of serotonin — it has many actions depending on where it is released and on which receptors it acts.

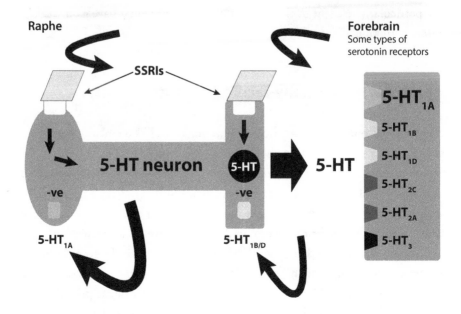

Figure 5: The serotonin neuron and synapse—
and where reuptake blockers work

Serotonin is known to be involved in a biological process that in other animal species goes back hundreds of millions of years, and with striking similarities to human mood changes. For example, lobsters and crayfish engage in battles over territory and when one loses the fight it adopts a body posture of defeat. This is due to a switching-off of serotonin in the nerves controlling the body posture. Social defeat in rodents and some primate species has also been shown to lead to lower levels of serotonin in the brain.

In humans, dieting (and other species low serotonin diets), particularly those that have low protein content have been shown to decrease serotonin function. This is especially evident in women because they have a faster metabolism of serotonin than men. As depressed people tend to eat less this relative deficit of serotonin may be a factor in perpetuating some cases of this disorder.

For a time before we had safe serotonin-promoting antidepressants such as the SSRIs, some depression research groups used to give dietary supplements of the immediate precursor of serotonin—5-HTP—to protect against depressive relapses. And although the primary precursor of serotonin, the amino-acid L-tryptophan, is not in itself an effective antidepressant, when added to antidepressant drugs that enhance serotonin it can boost their actions. This antidepressant effect of L-tryptophan can be quite powerful when it is given with drugs that block the breakdown of serotonin — the monoamine oxidase inhibitors (MAOIs) or with other medicine that enhance serotonin, e.g. lithium.

The MAOI class of antidepressant drug includes phenelzine and tranylcypromine and were the first true antidepressant drugs discovered. The history of their discovery is one of the most remarkable in psychiatry because they were originally, in the early-1950s, being tested as possible treatments for tuberculosis (TB). Astute doctors conducting the trial noted that although the TB wasn't improved by the test compounds the patients said they felt better in themselves, the drugs seemed to improve mood. Soon psychiatrists were testing them in patients with depression and anxiety and their treatment benefits became apparent. This was the first of many serendipitous discoveries of drug treatments in psychiatry. At the time serotonin had not been discovered but soon it was and the action of the MAOIs to prevent its breakdown determined. These drugs also prevent the breakdown of some other neurotransmitters particularly noradrenaline and dopamine and their antidepressant effect is likely to be due to an increased level of several of these in combination.

Serotonin enhancing drugs especially SSRIs are also potent anxiety-reducing agents particularly in disorders such as panic, post-traumatic stress disorder (PTSD) and social anxiety disorder. We now believe that the main action of increasing serotonin in the brain in these disorders and in depression is to enhance serotonin function at one subtype of the serotonin receptor called the 5-HT1A receptor. This is highly expressed in regions of the brain that regulate emotion such as the amygdala, insula and anterior cingulate cortex that we will discuss in *Chapter 8*. Here imaging studies in patients have found lower levels of these receptors so it is reasonable to assume that increasing serotonin with antidepressant medicines acts to compensate for this deficit.

Each serotonin receptor is coded by separate genes, but as each must have a protein sequence that serotonin can bind to, the determination of the human genome has made it possible to identify gene sequences that code for this region and so are common to all serotonin receptors. By this means 15 different receptors have been identified in different parts of the human genome and most of these are found in the brain. Currently we do not have selective molecular or chemical tools (drugs) to properly define each of their actions, but we do know that some of them have specific and important roles.

Only one of these serotonin receptor subtypes is an ion channel one, but it is one we know well from personal experience as it is the one that makes us vomit when we eat something toxic. This is the 5-HT3 receptor that is found in huge numbers on the vagus nerve (that connects the stomach with the brain). When we ingest a poison, serotonin is released from cells in the gut wall and blood. This activates these 5-HT3 receptors that then depolarise the vagus nerve making it send messages to the brain to induce vomiting and so clear the toxin from the body before more harm is done. One of the intriguing aspects of alcohol intoxication is that at some point people usually vomit. We now know this is due to high concentrations of alcohol stimulating the 5-HT3 receptor just like serotonin does. It may be that this is an important mechanism of defence against potentially fatal alcohol poisoning that could help explain the enduring use of alcohol by humans—as they often vomit before it kills them, they can repeat the experience again-and-again.

Unfortunately, the 5-HT3 receptor is also affected by potent anti-cancer treatments such as cisplatin. These cause the release of serotonin from cells in the gut and blood and this serotonin stimulates the 5-HT3 receptor leading to feelings of nausea, diarrhoea and in many cases severe vomiting. The discovery that the 5-HT3 receptor was responsible for serotonin-induced vomiting led to the development of selective blockers of this receptor such as ondansetron. These antagonists prevent serotonin stimulating these receptors and activating the vagus, and by this mechanism such 5-HT3 receptor antagonist drugs reduce chemotherapy-induced vomiting in cancer patients. They have become a major benefit to many patients for this reason.

Another type of serotonin receptor is the 5-HT1D. These are found on blood vessels particularly those feeding into the brain where they control blood flow. Migraine is a disabling syndrome of headaches and sensory changes such as lights around objects and zig-zag lines in vision. The exact cause of migraine is not known but these attacks are associated with increases in brain blood flow. Some 20 years ago several pharmaceutical companies decided to explore whether drugs targeting the 5-HT1D receptor might reduce this increase in blood flow and so limit migraine attacks. This proved to be a very viable approach and a new series of antimigraine agents called the tryptans have since been brought into medical practice. They can both prevent migraine attacks and stop them once started. This research also helped explain why older remedies for migraine such as ergotamine worked. These too act on serotonin receptors but in a less selective way than the tryptans.

Serotonin-directed ergot derivatives led to the discovery of psychedelic drugs such as LSD that act on another 5-HT receptor — the 5-HT2A receptor — in the brain. In a famous experiment Albert Hofmann, a chemist working for the Swiss pharmaceutical company Sandoz made a series of ergot derivatives as possible new treatments for disorders such as migraine. The 25th one in his new chemical series was the diethylamide version of the ergot derivative lysergic acid — hence the name LSD 25 = lysergic acid diethylamide. For a few years Hofmann let this compound rest on the shelf but in 1943 he accidentally ingested some and the psychedelic era was born. The effects he experienced were so out of the ordinary that they have become legend and the day he took it — April 20th that year — is now often celebrated on its anniversary. Hofmann reported profound alterations in the perception of light and colours and of space and time. His normal 30-minute cycle ride home seemed to take many hours.

When Hofmann reported these LSD-induced alterations of consciousness to his company bosses he persuaded them that LSD was a major breakthrough in brain science, and they made it available to researchers in many countries. In the 1950s and 1960s LSD was used by psychiatrists to mimic aspects of psychosis so they would understand their patients better, and to produce profound changes in the mental state of psychiatric patients that would lead to recovery from depression anxiety and addictions. In this period the National Institute of Health in the USA funded about 140 grants for LSD research that enrolled 40,000 patients and resulted in around 1,000 research publications. Overall, the results were quite positive revealing LSD to be a safe and effective treatment.

One of the most powerful examples was that of the founder of Alcoholics Anonymous, Bill Wilson. He became abstinent following a psychedelic experience and then pioneered the use of LSD to help alcoholics stop drinking. He believed that a single 'trip' could help them see that there were greater powers than alcohol in their lives. Wilson's enthusiasm and authority led to funding being made available for six trials of LSD to be conducted in alcoholics with impressive results. Most subjects were improved, and some gave up drinking permanently. Overall LSD was a more powerful treatment for alcohol addiction than any treatment before or since, even though it is only used once or twice in the course of therapy, because the effects are so enduring.

Pleased with these achievements Sandoz then developed another serotonin receptor agonist for therapeutic uses. This was psilocybin, the active ingredient in magic mushrooms. He worked out that psilocybin was like LSD in that both molecules had strong, structural resemblances to serotonin. Psilocybin has been used for millennia in many cultures across the world for personal growth and religious experiences and was then developed as a medicine with some success.

Given the clinical value of psychedelics, especially LSD, why don't we use them today? The answer is because they were made illegal in the 1960s. To some extent Wilson sowed the seeds of the destruction of LSD as a therapy when he introduced Aldous Huxley to it. Huxley was entranced by the experience of psychedelics and their ability to alter human consciousness and in the 1950s he wrote about this is his celebrated book, *The Doors of Perception*. This description of his trips and his insights into their nature and value soon became a classic and encouraged many others to explore the effects of psychedelics including the American psychologist and author Timothy Leary (1920–1996) who became very public enthusiasts.

These activists made repeated claims that psychedelics could change the world for the better, and these were welcomed and promulgated by the hippy anti-Vietnam war generation. The Establishments in the USA and UK saw the psychedelic movement as threatening the very essence of Western society which at the time was effectively at war with Russia and China in Vietnam. The USA Government then moved to curb psychedelic drug use by making such drugs illegal. This didn't stop recreational use but did completely stop their medical use. Since that time there have been just a couple of clinical studies with LSD and just a few with psilocybin, all in recent years. For over 40 years this field of inquiry was completely stopped which I believe is a clear form of censorship of research and clinical use of psychedelics and is arguably the worst censorship of science ever. It is one that needs to be rectified as soon as possible given the wide potential uses of psychedelics and their proven safety record.

How might psychedelics work to benefit people with mental illness? A major breakthrough has come from our research using brain imaging with these drugs. We found that both psilocybin and LSD fragment ongoing brain activity making it more random and less structured. We think this could disrupt the pathological repeated 'tramline' thinking that underlies conditions such as depression, addiction and obsessive-compulsive disorder (OCD) and so allow people to escape from this trap of repetitive negative thinking. They do this because these psychedelics stimulate the 5-HT2A receptor, and this receptor is widely distributed in the human cortex.

For reasons we don't understand, the human brain has more of these receptors than any other animal's brain and the most recently evolved parts of the cortex have the highest density of these receptors. This tells us that they are likely to be critical to human consciousness and our current hypothesis is that, when these receptors are stimulated, they mediate major vital changes in brain function allowing powerful and enduring changes in attitude and thinking to occur and persist. Psychedelics disrupt the normal repetitive routine processes of the brain so allowing new thoughts, ideas and even new approaches to problems to develop. Because serotonin is not involved in arousal and memory (these are the province of glutamate and GABA) the psychedelic experience is usually remembered very clearly by the person experiencing it, so the therapeutic effects persist and can be recalled for decades.

MDMA is another serotonin-acting drug that has had its therapeutic utility undermined by attempts to prevent its recreational use as the recreational rave drug ecstasy. MDMA works to release serotonin from the neuronal vesicles and, also, to block its reuptake. So it enhances serotonin function quite profoundly for a few hours. For reasons we don't yet understand the target effect of this released serotonin seems mainly to be in the emotional brain regions, and not the cortex, which is why MDMA is not a psychedelic.

As a chemical MDMA has been around for about 100 years, but it's fascinating effects on psychological processes wasn't revealed until the American biochemist, psychopharmacologist and author Alexander Shulgin (1925–2014) made and tried it out in the 1970s. He reported that MDMA had a profoundly different effect on him than any of the many other similar chemicals he had made and tested. He then shared some with his therapist wife Ann and together they realised that the experience of interpersonal warmth, insight and calmness that MDMA produces could have potential as a therapeutic agent. She shared it with friends who were psychotherapists conducting couples therapy and they found that a dose of MDMA could be of great benefit in helping them overcome the irritation and frustration with each other that years of marriage tend to produce. MDMA put them back to the time when they were actively in love and, when in this state, they were able to re-engage with each other in a much more positive and supportive manner, that continued well after the immediate effects of the drug had dissipated.

When used in this form of therapy MDMA was called 'empathy' by the therapists and its use raised no concerns with the authorities. Sadly, the suppliers of recreational drugs, who were looking for legal alternatives to amphetamine and cocaine, discovered the pleasurable effects of MDMA and related compounds. They started selling them for their energising as well as pro-love effects at clubs and raves. They also changed the name to 'ecstasy' to make it more sexy and so desirable.

By the 1980s ecstasy had become very popular with young people across the USA and Western Europe to the point where the media became aware of its use. They then started a hysterical campaign or 'moral panic' about this recreational use that was powered by scaremongering disinformation about its harms, with claims of brain damage and even deaths due to ecstasy use. Though these were greatly exaggerated the media exerted sufficient pressure on politicians to have the drug banned in the 1980s. This stopped the therapeutic use at a stroke, despite concerted rational pleadings for medical exemptions made to the authorities by the therapists. Since then a small group of committed researchers in the USA (the Multidisciplinary Association for Psychedelic Studies (MAPS)) has pushed for the resumption of clinical trials. Through charitable funding they have succeeded in conducting several trials in small groups of patients with resistant PTSD, with very good outcomes. Just two MDMA treatments as part of a psychotherapeutic package resulted in remarkable improvements in symptoms to the point where many previously untreatable patients were fully recovered. Now the USA Food and Drugs Agency and European Medicines Agency have agreed that because this research is targeting an area of medicine with great unmet need, a multi-centre trial can go ahead. This just reported (April 2021) as being successful and it looks like by the middle of this decade MDMA might once again be a medicine.

My own group has been working with MDMA as a possible treatment for alcoholism. We used the same regime as MAPS — just two 125 mg doses two weeks apart in the middle of a 14 weeks long psychotherapeutic programme. The results were as remarkable as those in PTSD — the vast majority of the alcoholic patients were able to stop, or markedly reduce, their drinking over the next nine months. The outcomes of our usual 14 weeks long treatment programmes are very much less good with less than a quarter of our patients staying sober at nine months. We now are looking for funding to do a larger placebo-controlled trial to replicate these exciting findings and if this works then MDMA might get approval as medicine for the treatment of alcoholism in a few years as well.

How MDMA works in PTSD and related disorders is still something of a mystery because its illegal status has meant that there have been almost no studies on its actions in the brain. The first whole-brain imaging study was conducted by my group in 2014 using fMRI. We found that a moderate (100mg) dose of MDMA had profound effects. In particular it decreased brain activity in the emotional brain circuits (see *Chapter 8*) especially the amygdala and hippocampus as well as decreasing connectivity between these two regions and the cortex.

We know from psychotherapy studies that the key to recovery in PTSD is for the patient to learn to confront the memory of the trauma for a period during which time they can exhaust (extinguish) the concomitant intense emotions that emerge alongside the memory because they were present at the original trauma. This learning to overcome the emotions of PTSD involves high level cortical regions suppressing the emergence of the emotions from lower regions such as the amygdala. Unfortunately, in many patients the emotions are so strong that they overwhelm the cortical control so that the patients never get an adequate duration of exposure to them to achieve extinction. We believe that our data showing MDMA helps suppress the brain regions controlling emotion explains why it can help patients control their emotional memories during therapy and so gain mastery of them.

Although few in number the serotonin neurons on the brain play many different roles in the brain with small specialised neuronal groups having different functions. Some seem to sense the levels of carbon dioxide in the blood and so generate fear responses and escape behaviour, so we don't suffocate. Others regulate eating behaviour by providing a sense of satiety of fullness. We see this in clinical eating disorders such as bulimia where high doses of the SSRI fluoxetine can attenuate the binge eating behaviour. This therapeutic action of fluoxetine is believed to be due to a combination of its increasing serotonin levels in the synaptic cleft and, also, having a direct action on a subtype of serotonin receptors that reduces appetite.

One of the most recently discovered roles of serotonin is in relation to touch and mood. Most of us enjoy a massage and often feel relaxed and happier after one. Babies respond wonderfully positively to being held and stroked, as do some adults; many others enjoy touching and stroking but don't have someone to do it with and so turn to companion animals for this pleasure. But why should physical touch impact on mood? The answer has been revealed in the form of a small group of serotonin neurons in the mid-brain that are activated by touching the skin. What's special about these neurons is that their outputs go directly to the part of the pre-frontal cortex (PFC) that controls mood and anxiety. So, touch has a fast track to the brain's high level mood centres which it turns on. We believe that other sensory stimuli such as warmth (e.g. a sauna) can also activate this set of neurons which can explain their mood-elevating properties too, and maybe even why so many of us like to go to hot sunny destinations on our vacations.

Other cultures have long understood the psychological value of heating the body and developed steam rooms (Turkish baths) saunas and 'sweat lodges' to achieve this end. More recently, Charles Raison and colleagues in the USA have developed a heating tent based on the sweat lodge principles and shown that periodic use of this can help people overcome depression. I suspect that the desire of increased touch that people get when they use MDMA is because this drug releases serotonin in this pathway, and touching magnifies this effect. We are trying to use brain imaging (see *Chapter 9*) to test this theory at present.

Noradrenaline — The fight or flight neurotransmitter

We have all had the experience of shaking with fear or anxiety—maybe after escaping a near miss car accident, or when someone has threatened us with violence or even attacked us. This shaking is mediated by another neurotransmitter called noradrenaline that works in the body as well as the brain. Noradrenaline is a neurotransmitter in part of the peripheral nervous system (the nerves outside of the brain and spinal cord) that controls blood pressure, sweating, muscle tone and pupil size, the so-called sympathetic nervous system. This is turned on when we are threatened and provides us with the physical resources to fight back—or to run away as fast as possible.

To do this noradrenaline is released from nerves that run from the spinal cord into blood vessels. When noradrenaline is released into them these vessels contract so increasing blood pressure. A large number of noradrenaline nerves go to the heart and when they release noradrenaline this increases the rate and the pumping power of the heart to provide the necessary increased blood flow to the muscles for fighting or fleeing. Noradrenaline also opens-up the airways of the lungs (the bronchi) so that more oxygen can get into the body and so power more muscle activity.

Noradrenaline is also a major neurotransmitter in terms of brain function. Although, as with serotonin and dopamine, there are relatively few noradrenaline neurons in the brain (about 200,000 compared to the billions of glutamate and GABA ones), the massively branched structure of their axons means that each noradrenaline neuron can innervate millions of other types of neuron. In this way noradrenaline can modulate activity across large brain regions and set the tone for neuronal activities and behaviour patterns.

One of the main functions of noradrenaline in the brain is to maintain arousal. Noradrenaline is one of the neurotransmitters that keep us awake and facilitates sustained attention and concentration. The activity of noradrenaline neurons is switched-off during sleep and they turn on as we wake-up. Many years ago, I was researching idazoxan, a new kind of drug designed to increase brain noradrenaline and treat depression. I was part of a group that took it for a few weeks to find out what it did to sleep and hormones. We found it did affect the brain in a way consistent with an increase in noradrenaline. It was especially effective in getting me awake in the mornings, as soon as I woke, I was up and ready to go. This is more evidence that brain noradrenaline drives arousal and wakefulness.

As with most other neurotransmitters, noradrenaline can act on a number of different receptors. The action of noradrenaline to maintain arousal and attention in the brain is mediated through the alpha1 and alpha2 subtypes. The effect of noradrenaline to increase blood pressure and heart rate in the cardiovascular system is through the beta receptor subtypes. Drugs that block beta receptors (so called beta blockers) were one of the first pharmacologically designed and targeted treatments for high blood pressure (hypertension) and have saved millions of lives from heart failure and strokes in the five decades since they were developed.

Drugs that block noradrenaline alpha1 receptors also work in the peripheral circulatory system to lower blood pressure, but they have major effects in the brain too—they reduce attention and concentration and make people very sleepy. For these reasons they are no longer used to control blood pressure. However, one of these old drugs, prazosin, has recently been resurrected because the once-adverse effect of sedation can now be turned to therapeutic use in helping to suppress nightmares in conditions such as PTSD where they can be very disturbing and sleep disrupting.

Nightmares are not caused by the release of noradrenaline but the emotions they precipitate, despite occurring when people are asleep, they lead to the noradrenaline neurons becoming activated. This then wakes the person from sleep, so they are made aware of, and are thus distressed by, the traumatic memory yet again. Blocking alpha noradrenaline receptors makes waking during nightmares less likely so patients suffer less. We shall see later that blocking beta receptors can also be useful in reducing some fear states.

One conceptualisation of anxiety is of an excessive or maladaptive level of arousal, a concept developed about a century ago in the now famous Yerkes-Dodson curve—see *Figure 6.*

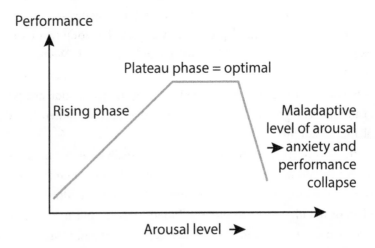

Figure 6: Arousal anxiety and performance—Yerkes-Dodson curve

We need to be aroused to perform, an experience we have daily when waking-up and getting ready for work. Many of us use stimulants: drugs (tea, coffee) or nicotine (tobacco) to move our arousal level up this slope. As our arousal levels rise, we perform better until we reach the optimal or plateau state. But if arousal continues to increase then we can be tipped-over into a state of excessive arousal where performance falls off, this is then maladaptive. We call it an anxiety state.

If anxiety occurs suddenly then we call it a 'panic attack' and if it is more chronic and ongoing it is labelled 'generalised anxiety disorder.' People in this over-aroused state inevitably find their cognitive abilities are profoundly impaired. Students getting a panic attack in an exam can forget what they have learned and even what they are supposed to be doing so they just freeze.

Noradrenaline is thought to be the major neurotransmitter involved in this increase in arousal and then in anxiety (see earlier in this chapter). The psychological effects from its release in the brain are accompanied by its release in the periphery which leads to the heart beating faster, the stomach churning ('butterflies in the tummy'), pains in the chest and in some cases sweating. Together these contribute to the range of symptoms seen in anxiety disorders.

Often the physical symptoms are more distressing to the person than the anxiety, so they worry that the increase in heart rate means they are going to have a heart attack or butterflies in the tummy means they have cancer. They often seek medical help for these illness fears and present to the emergency services or to casualty departments where medics use a lot of resources proving they are not physically ill. It has been estimated that in some centres, over half of all people presenting with chest pains are having a panic attack rather than a cardiac event. Many of them get expensive, dangerous and unnecessary investigations such as cardiac catheters, so a proper, early diagnosis can benefit everyone.

Why some people go over the arousal curve more readily than others is still being researched but one theory is that their noradrenaline neurons are deficient in the usual negative feedback processes (the pre-synaptic alpha2 receptor) that work to prevent excessive noradrenaline activity. Drugs that block anxiety and panic attacks often make this feedback more efficient so stabilise noradrenaline neuron firing.

Strangely we can sometimes upset this negative feedback to our advantage for example in cases of depression where there may be a deficiency of noradrenaline. By blocking the pre-synaptic alpha2 receptor we can increase noradrenaline in the brain and some current antidepressant drugs work in this way (mianserin, mirtazapine). Other antidepressant drugs can increase noradrenaline by blocking its reuptake (reboxetine, nortriptyline, desipramine) and some serotonin reuptake blockers also block noradrenaline reuptake as well (venlafaxine, duloxetine, amitriptyline, clomipramine, imipramine). In severe cases of depression, we sometimes use both sorts—the pre-synaptic alpha2 receptor blockers and the reuptake blockers together to maximise the impact on noradrenaline to give the best antidepressant effect possible.

A paradox still to be resolved is why don't these drugs increase anxiety when increasing noradrenaline. One explanation is that they also block other receptors such as the histamine 1 receptor that produces a counteracting anxiolytic effect. Another is that the rate of rise of noradrenaline is quite slow with these drugs and takes place over the course of many days so the brain has time to adapt. It is sudden surges in noradrenaline that tend to lead to anxiety and panic.

Dopamine — The get up and go neurotransmitter

A close relative of noradrenaline is dopamine, another small amine chemical that acts as a neurotransmitter in some parts of the brain particularly those relating to movement and planning. Dopamine started life as a precursor to the neurotransmitter noradrenaline and then became utilised as a neurotransmitter much later in evolution. Probably because it was the last of the three amine neurotransmitters (serotonin-noradrenaline-dopamine) to evolve, dopamine has a much more localised distribution in the brain than the other two. Serotonin and noradrenaline neurons spread their axons over all of the brain whereas those of the dopamine neurons are limited to the basal ganglia where it regulates fluid movements, in the emotional brain (limbic system) where it has a role in mood and motivation, and in the prefrontal cortex where it helps maintain attention and concentration: see *Figure 7*.

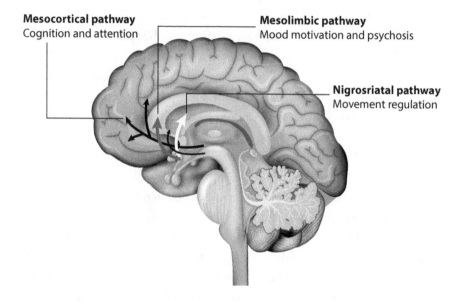

Mesocortical pathway
Cognition and attention

Mesolimbic pathway
Mood motivation and psychosis

Nigrosriatal pathway
Movement regulation

Figure 7: Distribution of dopamine neuronal systems in the human brain

But in the field of human brain science dopamine has a very special place as it was the first neurotransmitter to be identified as being involved in a human brain disorder — Parkinson's disease.

The story of the identification of dopamine deficiency as the cause of Parkinson's disease began in the 1950s. Dopamine had just been discovered as a neurotransmitter and then post-mortem studies of the brains of people with Parkinson's disease showed a profound deficit of the neurons that make dopamine. This led to a remarkable new therapeutic approach — replacing the missing neurotransmitter by giving its precursor L-DOPA, which in the brain is turned into dopamine.

The story of the discovery of L-DOPA therapy was immortalised in the 1970s book *Awakenings* by Oliver Sacks in which he explains how he did this successfully in a group of patients in New York. This is one of the great narratives in medicine which explains why it was turned into a play 'A Kind of Alaska' by Harold Pinter and then the feature film 'Awakenings' that starred Robin Williams and Robert de Niro. These all tell the story of a group of patients who had seemingly untreatable brain damage caused by an influenza virus that produced encephalitis lethargica. Their brain damage was sustained in the 1920s after they contracted the Great Influenza (often but wrongly called the Spanish Flu). For nearly 40 years they were usually immobile or very slowed down with limited speech, emotional and cognitive responses, as if in a kind of persistent sleep or coma (described by one as 'a kind of Alaska,' hence the name of the play). However, when given L-DOPA they rapidly woke-up (hence the book's title *Awakenings*) and began to move and speak normally as the deficit of dopamine in their brain was replenished.

This was the first demonstration that a brain disorder could be caused by a depletion of a neurotransmitter and be treated by its replacement. It provided the paradigm for subsequent research into other brain disorders and the invention of new treatments. These efforts have yielded many insights into a range of different brain disorders, e.g. Huntingdon's and Alzheimer's diseases. It has also led to the development of some novel treatments, e.g. the discovery of the loss of acetylcholine in Alzheimer's disease led to treatments such as donepezil and galantamine that enhance it. The SSRIs were developed partly because of evidence of serotonin deficiency in the brains of people who died with depression.

The discovery of dopamine and the subsequent elucidation of how it is produced in the brain led to an understanding of how most neurotransmitters are manufactured and regulated—see *Chapter 1*.

As we saw earlier many neurons have developed sophisticated processes to collect neurotransmitters back into the releasing neuron so they can be re-used, the reuptake sites or transporters. These reuptake sites on dopamine neurons are the target site for many drugs and medicines such as the antidepressant and anti-smoking agent bupropion (Wellbutrin, Zyban). This compound acts to partially block them so increases dopamine levels in the synapse (*Figure 5*). This leads to a positive effect of mood to lift depression. The increase in dopamine also protects against the drop off in dopamine that contributes to the low mood and cravings for nicotine that occur during tobacco withdrawal and lead so many people to a return to smoking.

Amphetamines, cocaine and related stimulants (e.g. crack cocaine and crystal meth) also block dopamine reuptake and in some cases reverse the pump leading to a large increase in synaptic dopamine concentrations. This explains the increase in energy and drive with, in some cases, extreme pleasure and euphoria. These experiences can mimic mania and precipitate it in some people so predisposed.

Animal studies have shown that if these drugs are taken repeatedly at frequent intervals and at high doses adaptive downward changes in the dopamine system develop in an attempt to compensate for this excess stimulation—this is called 'tolerance.' These adaptive brain changes mean that when a person stops using the stimulant they go into in a state of withdrawal with a relative dopamine deficiency which is associated with low mood, irritability, listlessness, etc. Such withdrawal states are very unpleasant and often provoke the user to go back on the stimulant to reverse them. But repeated stimulation of dopamine release doesn't always lead to tolerance. In some neurons paradoxical increases in dopamine function are seen, the so-called sensitisation effect. Together these changes can lead to animals becoming addicted to these drugs and using them compulsively, and we believe that elements of human addiction to stimulants have a similar biochemical basis. However not everyone who takes strong stimulants, even crack cocaine or crystal, gets addicted so there must be other processes in play.

It is important to realise that not every drug that increases dopamine in the brain has the propensity to be addictive. We have already mentioned the anti-addictive efficacy of bupropion (Zyban) for tobacco smoking. Other dopamine enhancing drugs such as methylphenidate (Ritalin) and amphetamine are used to treat the attentional deficits seen in patients with attention deficit hyperactivity disorder (ADHD). These are not addictive when used properly as they only slowly increase dopamine levels. Addiction to stimulants is most likely when fast increases in dopamine are produced, and this can be encouraged by injecting drugs IV (e.g. cocaine) or by smoking them (crack, crystal). These two routes of administration get drugs into the brain in a couple of minutes whereas medication taken orally requires 30 mins or more to be absorbed.

There is more to the dopamine system than reuptake sites and stimulants. Some of the most important drugs in the history of medicine are blockers of dopamine receptors. These are used to treat schizophrenia and mania and are called neuroleptics or antipsychotics. The first one to be discovered was chlorpromazine which was developed in the early-1950s as a sedative antihistamine -like drug similar to phenergan.

In those days there were no specific treatments for schizophrenia so patients were locked in asylums and sedated with drugs as required. The French pair of doctors Jean Delay and Pierre Denicker were trying out this new sedative chlorpromazine in their wards and they noted something quite special, rather than simply sedating patients, chlorpromazine made them less psychotic. It reduced their symptoms of schizophrenia. They quickly shared this amazing discovery with the world and coined the term neuroleptic to explain the effect it had to calm the schizophrenic mind. Since then, many drugs that reduce the symptoms of schizophrenia have been discovered and as a class they are now called 'antipsychotics.'

Chlorpromazine instigated the first pharmacological revolution in psychiatry. Until 1952 there had been a year-on-year increase in the number of people (often young men) held in asylums because they had schizophrenia. After 1952 the numbers began to fall and have continued to do so ever since. Chlorpromazine helped millions of people leave the asylums and move back to their homes or into the community because they were no longer severely mentally-ill. So long as they continued to take their medication, they were well enough to function outside of hospital. But the discovery of chlorpromazine was pure serendipity, astute clinicians noting that it worked. At that time no-one had any idea why or how. It took a further five years for that to become clear, and this required the discovery of dopamine in the brain.

Once dopamine was identified in the brain then studies began to explore how it was made, and the amino-acid L-DOPA was identified as the precursor. If animals were given L-DOPA then dopamine concentrations in the brain rose—which is why it was used (as already mentioned) to treat Parkinson's disease when the dopamine deficit was discovered. The breakdown of dopamine was then worked out to be via the mechanism of action (MAO) enzyme we have already described in relation to serotonin degradation.

When in rats MAO is blocked and L-DOPA is then given, a state of manic hyper-activity ensues that looks rather like that produced by stimulants such as amphetamine. Moreover, the combination of amphetamine plus L-DOPA increased activity even more suggesting that amphetamine might work through enhancing dopamine.

The key breakthrough in understanding chlorpromazine came when, in 1957, Arvid Carlsson working in Sweden found that it could block this state of stimulant-induced hyper-activity, suggesting it was a dopamine antagonist. This theory was finally proved in 1974 by the group of Phil Seeman in Canada who developed a means to measuring dopamine receptors in the brain and showed that chlorpromazine and other antipsychotic drugs bound to this receptor, so blocking the effects of dopamine. However, long before this discovery was made the ability of chlorpromazine to stop amphetamine induced hyper-activity was utilised as an assay to screen for other drugs that did the same.

Many of the drugs we use today were identified by this bio-assay process. For example, at the same time Carlsson was making his Nobel Prize-winning discoveries, a possible role for dopamine in psychosis was inferred by the pharmacist Paul Janssen in Belgium. He noted that road racing cyclists were commonly becoming paranoid as a result of using amphetamines to enhance their performance (this was allowed at that time, doping bans in the sport only came in the 1960s). He then set out to find a dopamine blocking drug and synthesised haloperidol, which became an extremely popular antipsychotic that is still used today in the treatment of both schizophrenia and mania.

The fact that antipsychotic drugs blocked the actions of dopamine led to the theory that schizophrenia and mania are due to an excess production and release of dopamine. In the case of mania this seems to be the case since so many of the symptoms of this disorder, such as euphoria, hyper-activity, loss of sleep and speeded thinking can be mimicked in normal people by stimulants. The case of schizophrenia is more complex as only the paranoia is reliably produced by stimulants and then only when used to excess in binges. However, PET brain scanning (*Chapter 9*) has shown that about half of people with this disorder do have an overactive dopamine system, which explains why dopamine blockers are helpful in them. But the other group of patients may have some other as yet unidentified brain disorder, and these do not respond well at all to these medicines.

Endorphins — From pain to pleasure

Popular opinion has it that the endorphins are the source of pleasure. It is widely believed that these neurotransmitters are released under circumstances that lead to a feeling of being high, e.g. after sex and exercise (the so-called 'runner's high'). The reality is a little different with good evidence that endorphins are released when people are in pain. This makes sense as they act on the (mu) opioid receptor that is also the target of pain killers such as morphine and codeine. In other words, the endorphins are the brain's natural analgesics that are mimicked by analgesic drugs such as morphine that are derived from opium found in some species of poppies (hence the term opioid).

Why the opium poppy should manufacture a substance like opium is not really known but we think that many plants make potent chemicals such as opium, nicotine and atropine, to deter predators such as insects or mammals. These chemicals have evolved to act on receptors already present in the eater's brain. A few take the opposite view that the brain receptors that are sensitive to plant products evolved to allow us to benefit from eating substances such as opium or psilocybin (the ingredient in magic mushrooms). Maybe both are to some extent correct.

There is some emerging evidence that endorphins may play a role in pleasure in that they can be released by drugs such as alcohol and amphetamine and the greater the extent of this endorphin release the more pleasure is experienced. This mediation of some of the actions of alcohol by endorphins has led to the development of new treatments for alcoholism, specifically the opioid receptor blockers naltrexone and nalmefene.

Naltrexone is a licensed treatment for alcohol addiction, for assisting people in their maintenance of abstinence as part of a planned programme of alcoholism treatment. When taken on a daily basis it seems to work by helping those who are abstinent but then have a temporary lapse in self-control and take a couple of drinks from losing complete control and suffering a fully-blown relapse to regular heavy drinking. This discovery led to the development of nalmefene (also known by the trade name Selincro). This is the first medicine to be approved to help drinkers with alcohol problems control the amount they drink.

Most of us will know of someone who wishes to drink normally but once they start can't control their intake, and they go on a binge or a 'bender' and get very drunk. Time-and-time-again they set out with the good intention of just having a couple of drinks as their friends do. But once they have had these a switch seems to be thrown in their brain and they then lose self-control and drink much more alcohol than they intended. The next day they may or may not be hungover but almost always they are regretful of their loss-of-control and vow never to do it again, but of course they do.

Nalmefene when used as part of a treatment programme with appropriate psychological support can reduce the number of heavy drinking days (binges) in people with alcohol dependence by up to 40 per cent over placebo. This is associated with improvements in mental wellbeing and liver health. I call nalmefene a 'drinking regulator' and believe in it, and hopefully other drugs that in future will be developed to help people regulate their drinking. If they are this will have considerable potential to reduce the extreme social and health damage caused by alcohol in the UK.

Until nalmefene there were no medications to help people regulate their drinking; the only approved treatment options were based on abstinence. But abstinence is a tough path to follow in countries like ours where the vast majority of people drink. It singles out the non-drinker as someone very different and this can be quite uncomfortable, even stigmatising. Moreover, most people with alcohol problems want to be able to control their drinking and enjoy alcohol in moderation like the majority of us do.

We do not yet know how blockade of opioid receptors by nalmefene or naltrexone effects changes in drinking control. It may be that it reduces the pleasures of alcohol consumption, or it may improve the ability of the brain to control its desires. Certainly, alcohol leads to endorphin release in the brain areas responsible for these behaviours, so by blocking these actions opioid receptor antagonists may prevent loss of control over drinking.

Endorphins are not the only endogenous opioid receptor neurotransmitters. Another is called dynorphin and this appears to be the alter-ego of endorphins; whereas they can lead to pleasure, dynorphin induces distress. Why the brain has a distress-inducing system is a matter of some speculation, but it may be to help the brain learn to avoid painful or threatening circumstances. It appears that dynorphins work to decrease the release of dopamine in the pleasure centres of the brain so leading to a form of depression. This would then predict that antagonists of dynorphin receptors might offset the effects of stress and so improve mood and several such compounds are now showing promise in clinical trials for depression.

CHAPTER 3

The Tower of Complexity — How the Brain is Organized

E veryone with sight has seen multiple images of the brain with its cau-
liflower-like complexly-folded surface. This is the cerebral cortex, the
highest and most recently evolved part of the brain and that part which
gives us the remarkable capacity for thought and communication that distinguishes us from all other species.

The evolution of the cortex is thought to be the most rapid evolutionary
event in history, with an increase in volume of several-fold emerging over a
few thousand generations. What drove this is not known but some social psy-
chologists believe that it was a result of social interactions in our early tribal
groups increasing brain functionality and then leading to more growth. Others
believe that the use of serotonin stimulating plants such as magic mushrooms
promoted brain growth.

Genetic factors are likely also relevant and a gene that may be implicated has
recently been discovered in mice. However, so great was the growth spurt of
the human cerebral cortex that in order for all of it to fit into the skull it has to
be crumpled up like a page of paper being crushed into a ball in the hand. In
fact, it's two rather oval-shaped balls because there are two sides (hemispheres)
of the cortex that connect via a massive neuronal pathway in the middle of the
brain called the 'corpus callosum.'

For centuries observations on people with brain injuries and tumours gave
us insights into what the different parts of the brain do. The cortex is where
much of the higher functions of the brain take place. Different regions of the
cortex do different things (see *Figure 8*). So, the back (occipital) cortex is where

we see and store visual memories. The upper side regions are where touch and movement are located, whereas lower down are the hearing regions. The frontal region (frontal lobe) was for a long time thought redundant since the effects of damage there are much less apparent than those from damage to the movement or speaking regions that are so commonly affected by strokes.

In fact, there are other parts of the brain long known to have less obvious effects from damage. These were called the 'silent' brain regions, as opposed to those where damage was obvious, the so-called 'eloquent' cortex because damage there had clear manifestations. We now know from more sophisticated studies particularly using neuroimaging that these 'silent' regions are actively involved in processes such as thinking and planning and comparing and reflecting rather than movement and processing sensory inputs. Indeed, they are where our special human consciousness originates.

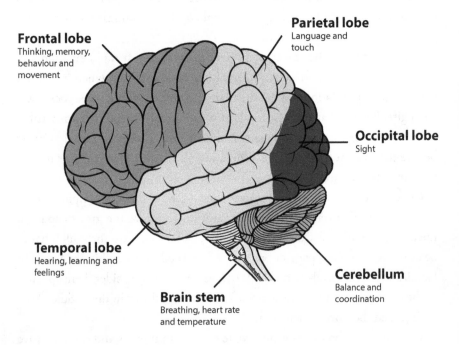

Figure 8: Brain regions and functions—Outside view of one hemisphere

Accidental insights into brain organization — The strange case of Phineas Gage

The frontal lobe was the last to reveal its secrets and did so in the remarkable case of a USA railwayman — Phineas Gage. In the 1800s he worked as an explosives expert blowing rocks out of the way to build cuttings for those who laid the railway tracks in New England. Gage's job was to drill holes in the rock then pound explosive deep into each hole with a long rod of iron (a tamping rod). One day he made a mistake and the explosive detonated as he was tamping it in, the rod blew out of the hole like a rocket and went right through the front of his head, in at the eye socket and out at the top of his head. Remarkably he didn't die then and there and perhaps even more remarkably his brain did not get infected. In fact, Gage seemed to make a full recovery, the wounds healed and he was able to go back to work. But then his life began to fall apart, because he was a different person, his personality had changed, and not for the better.

Contemporary descriptions of Gage record that before the accident he was a pious God-fearing family man. Afterwards he became a womanising drunkard who eventually was kicked out of his family and lost his job. The tamping iron had dramatically changed his personality and we now know this was because, as it flew through his skull, it destroyed a large chunk of the frontal lobe. From examples like Phineas Gage, we can deduce that this frontal part of the brain is responsible for aspects of personality such as reliability, responsibility and even being God-fearing. The frontal lobe is the site of our self-control.

Similar forms of frontal brain damage are common in other traumatic injuries to the head, particularly from motorcycle accidents. Even in my own career I have come across colleagues whose personalities and so lives have been fundamentally changed by such events. Much more often I have seen it happen as a result of alcohol and other drugs that can also damage this brain region, both directly and as a result of drug-induced fights and falls leading to traumatic damage to the front of the brain.

One particular example got me into a lot of trouble with the UK Government when I was the UK Drug Czar, as chair of the Advisory Council on the Misuse of Drugs (ACMD). It related to the case of a middle-aged woman who had incurred significant personality changes from brain damage that resulted from falling off her horse. She had become disinhibited, inattentive and impulsive to the point where she could no longer hold down her job. Worse her husband left her, taking their children with him because she had become so difficult to live with—they were always arguing—and in reality, she was no longer the same woman he had married.

She consulted me in my capacity as an expert psychopharmacologist who had experience of treating other patients with personality change produced by brain damage. In some cases, the careful use of stimulants such as Ritalin or amphetamine can help reduce the attentional and behavioural problems that can result from frontal lobe damage. I tried these in my patient but with only limited success and it became clear her life had been irrevocably changed by her fall, in the same way as had Gage's life. This woman's misfortune got me interested in the question of how common was brain damage from horse-riding, so I did what all researchers do when a question arises, an internet literature search. To my amazement, because I had allowed, indeed encouraged, my two daughters to ride, I found a number of papers detailing the harms of horse-riding. These range from death to brain damage and of course fractured spines and limbs. Even Superman (i.e. the American actor Christopher Reeve) died from the complications of breaking his back falling from a horse. In the USA there are several thousand deaths per year from horse-riding accidents and in the UK around 50, with eventing and jumping being the most dangerous riding activity. The dangers of horse-riding are well known around the world and the Italians have a saying for it, *'uomo a cavallo, sepoltura aperta!'* which translates as 'Man on horse, grave open!'

Despite these risks millions of people ride and many know personally of other riders who have been injured or died. A colleague of mine (partially) broke their neck several times falling from their horse yet still rides. Perhaps the most remarkable example of riding in the face of damage is the *Times* journalist Melanie Reid. She broke her neck and back falling from her horse and was immobile for months and in severe pain and muscle spasm. But has since got back on a horse even though her back is held together by a steel frame. She does this because:

'It's a passion, a thrill, a love affair. Because it brings that sense of being alive, properly alive in a way there is an implicit contract with the devil—you know it's dangerous but you are willing to accept and suffer the consequences.'

But when she gets back on her horse her back goes into spasm as she has stopped the anti-spasmodic benzodiazepine drug clonazepam for fear of dependence. A strange example of risk comparisons.

Still Melanie's desire to ride overcomes her fear of becoming dependent on the clonazepam so she goes back on the horse because, 'If it is a choice between riding a horse and taking a strong drug then there's no debate.' Her experience and account of her feelings tells us that she is addicted to riding. Based on cases like hers I invented the term Equasy (short for Equine Addiction Syndrome) and wrote a paper comparing the harms of Equasy with those of another recreational pursuit with a similar name, ecstasy (i.e. MDMA).

From my research on their relative risks and harms I concluded Equasy was more harmful than ecstasy. I thought this was an important comparison because at the time the ACMD was reviewing the classification of MDMA which was then in the most dangerous class A category, and I thought that comparing it with something as common and accepted as horse-riding might help the Government come to a more rational decision on its harms. I was wrong! This conclusion did not go down at all well with the Government at the time and I was ticked off by the Home Secretary, Jacqui Smith, for insulting families who had lost members from horse-riding. For reasons I still don't understand I was also attacked by the horse-riding community, presumably because they prefer not to know the risks they take every time they mount a horse.

Alcohol — A reversible way to switch-off the frontal cortex

Thankfully, few of us will ever suffer brain damage to our frontal lobe. But many if not most of us will have experienced to some extent the impact of changing frontal lobe function in a transient way. Most usually, this is when we have been drunk and done things that are quite out of character, perhaps getting into a fight or making a fool of ourselves with someone we fancied but who didn't reciprocate?

Alcohol in moderate doses produces a temporary blunting of frontal lobe function. Other drugs, particularly stimulants such as cocaine and crystal meth(amphetamine), can produce even more extreme disinhibition of frontal lobe activity. In practice these disinhibiting effects on the frontal lobes are the reason why most people take these drugs in the first place — they want to lose control and escape their responsibilities. The same is true for alcohol, which gives the lie to the drinks industry's call to 'drink responsibly,' since most of us drink to get a transient escape from responsibility! Some prostitutes and others who have to engage in behaviour they find repellent and disgusting use drugs to dampen down their frontal lobe's attempts to resist the behaviour. Child soldiers in Africa were commonly given strong stimulants to deaden their moral resistance to killing. The concept of *in-vino veritas* (in wine truth) developed from similar observations.

Most of us use our frontal lobes all the time to regulate what we say to and about other people. We know that in many cases if we let our true feelings out then it's likely that offence will be taken. Alcohol impairs this ability to self-regulate by dampening frontal lobe function, so it's harder to mislead others — we are more likely to tell the truth, or at least expose our feelings and desires, when drunk. Some would go further and say that we are more likely to show our true character too, but this is more questionable since alcohol affects many other more primitive brain regions.

The ancient Greeks knew of this lie-preventing effect of alcohol, and this is why they preferred to have their senators debate when under 'the influence' as this made it harder for them to dissemble or lie. The Ancient Persians are reputed to have used alcohol in the evening when trying to develop creative solutions to problems, but wisely would not act on these until after discussing them again the next morning when sober!

CHAPTER 4

The Vital Role of Subconscious Processing

The cortex (as described in the previous chapter) is the final target of sensory inputs from eyes, ears, touch, sensors, etc. and it integrates these with memories and plans to develop the most appropriate responses, often with conscious awareness. However, most of what the body needs to do takes place at lower levels in the central nervous system (CNS). It is important to react fast to certain dangers—you don't want to have to make a conscious decision to pull your hand out of a fire—you just want it to happen as fast as possible to minimise tissue damage and pain.

These fast protective actions take place as reflexes, below conscious control. Their inputs and outputs are hard wired in the lower parts of the brain and in the spinal cord and are (necessarily) insulated from conscious input. Many happen without the person even being aware of them. An eye blink, to prevent a piece of dust getting into the eye for instance takes place literally 'in the blink of an eye' usually without any conscious awareness. Of course, when this fails to stop the eye getting irritated then we are very aware of it.

If you step on a tack your leg retracts before you feel the pain, because the retraction takes place in the spinal cord but the pain isn't perceived until the nerve sensations reach the brain. In fact, a remarkable amount of activity occurs at the spinal level. Much of the process of walking is generated by spinal circuits, hence in people with spinal cord transections electrical stimulation of the spinal cord itself, below the damaged part, can reinstate walking. The example of standing on a tack shows another ability of the spinal cord. As you lift one leg away from the tack the muscles in the other leg are made to contract appropriately by neurons in the spinal cord, so you don't fall over!

These processes of reciprocal actions between neurons are a fundamental feature of the CNS and so are seen at all levels up to and including the cortex. There are at least four, and in the case of the visual system many more, layers of processing neurons between the outside world and our awareness of it. For example, the touch of a finger is detected by sensors just under the outer layers of the skin. These activate the neurons attached to them so sending a message to the spinal cord. Here the first stage of processing occurs when these sensory inputs activate another set of neurons that carry the information up to the brain. But in the spinal cord other local neurons are activated that alter the input of other sense detectors and give priority to the touch signal. This we see in everyday life when we are in pain and rub the offending limb as this activates these touch inputs that dominate the pain ones, a process called 'sensory gating.'

Traditional interventions such as acupuncture work in the same way. I once had a ring stolen from my finger during a conversation through a train window in India. At the time I couldn't work out how the thief managed to get it off of my finger without my feeling anything, but on reflection realised he had been touching my upper arm on that side so blocking out feelings from my finger lower down the limb.

Another level of complexity in the spinal cord comes because sensory inputs can be controlled by neurons that descend from the brain. These can magnify or minimise the function and explain how the brain can overcome pain when in great need to do so, e.g. when in a battle many people suffer wounds that they don't notice until the urgency of the fighting is over. Indian fakirs can walk on hot charcoal without suffering pain because they have trained their brain to deny access of the pain fibre inputs to consciousness. Such powerful overrides from descending neuronal pathways help explain why yogis expert in deep meditation can slow their heart rate to levels only otherwise seen in hibernating animals.

These descending pathways can enhance as well as inhibit ascending function which explains seemingly inexplicable phenomena such as seen in conversion disorders (what used to be called hysteria). These physiological changes such as intestinal bloating and flushing of the limbs were (and in some churches are still) interpreted as possession by God or by the Devil as in the classic descriptions of *The Devils of Loudon* by Aldous Huxley.

Moving from the spinal cord into the brain another bridging point is met—the thalamus (see *Figures 8* and *9*). This is in effect an evolutionary, very old mini-brain that can integrate and provide reflex responses to sensory inputs in the absence of the higher regions such as cortex. Primitive vertebrates (animals with a spinal cord) all have a thalamus equivalent that serves as their 'brain.' In the case of fish it does enough to keep them swimming towards food and away from predators, as it can integrate touch and movement sensory inputs with hearing and visual and smell inputs. In humans the sensory neurons synapse in the thalamus and the next neurons project into the sensory cortex where the touch is 'felt.' But from the thalamus other neuronal outputs go to other parts of the brain as part of the process of integration of inputs and outputs that are vital for life as we know it. As we have already seen, some go back down to the spinal cord to modify inputs, while some go to the other sensory input systems such as seeing and hearing so providing for an integrated assessment of the environment. Others go to activate the brain's arousal systems to ensure that there is an optimal level of wakefulness in responses to threatening stimuli and proper attention is given to it.

Once the touch sensation hits the cortex (*Figures 8* and *9*) then a further set of complex interactions takes place. The sensory cortex communicates with other parts of sensory cortex (vision, hearing, taste smell, etc.) to create a schema of what the touch input relates to—it is just a local touch to the finger as from picking up a cup of tea, or is it that the person is about to pour boiling water into the cup? In either case appropriate movements need to be initiated, whether opening the mouth to drink or steadying the hands holding cup and kettle. These movements are planned in frontal parts of the brain (the supplementary motor areas) that then direct the motor cortex to programme the neuronal outputs to make them occur. But all the time these motor outputs produce alterations in sensory inputs that are re-evaluated by the brain and used to continually refine and optimise the motor outputs to produce the remarkable precision of movement that we and other animals have.

In other words, the brain and spinal cord are a series of input and output neuronal feedback loops. Primary descending outputs determine movement of muscles to allow us to move to seek food and drink, protect ourselves, locate mates, build homes, and defend our families. In many animals they also include the making of sounds to warn tribal members of threat or to scare off predators.

In humans this sound-making motor activity occurs in the muscles of the larynx and pharynx that allow us to speak. But the human brain has developed a remarkable sophistication in terms of the motor programmes of these muscles so that a unique range of sounds we call speech and music can be produced.

Ensuring the optimal production of movements requires engagement of secondary brain circuits, called the basal ganglia, that also work as a series of neuronal loops. These structures receive massive neuronal inputs containing the neurotransmitter dopamine, which is critical for movement. When dopamine neurons are destroyed, patients are left with encephalitis lethargica, a severe form of Parkinson's disease. Lesser degrees of dopamine loss result in motor slowness and often tremor. The tremor we now know is due to disruption of the normal reciprocal neuronal connections between the different parts of the basal ganglia that can in some cases be rectified by surgically implanting electrodes into the brain to normalise the aberrant feedback (the technique is called deep brain stimulation).

Higher-level cortical functions also involve a massive series of feedback loops across the cortex—from sensory input regions to planning regions to motor regions and back again. In later chapters we shall see how these can be disrupted by psychedelic drugs to help treat psychiatric disorders such as obsessive compulsive disorder (OCD). But we can also see deficits in these internal feedback systems contributing to altered mental states.

A good example of what happens when feedback within the cortex goes awry is with auditory hallucinations (hearing voices) in schizophrenia. When we want to speak, a specialised part of the frontal lobe cortex generates the content of what we want to say. This then sends messages to the motor speech centre to organize the muscle activity in the mouth larynx and diaphragm to produce the right sounds. But in addition, this frontal lobe region also sends messages to the hearing centre to shut it down, so the brain doesn't get confused by hearing what it is saying.

In schizophrenia the work of the UK neuroscientist Chris Frith has shown that this internal shut-down system doesn't work adequately, so people who suffer this awful syndrome in effect 'hear' their own speech-thoughts which they misinterpret as other peoples' voices. In extreme cases of schizophrenia, the voices are heard clearly as coming from outside the head, but as treatment begins to work, they gradually lose this clear sense of them being from outside and they become heard more 'inside the head' until they can in some cases disappear.

The process whereby voices become heard is not clear but we know that dopamine is involved in some way as the antipsychotic drugs that reduce these hallucinations work by blocking subtypes of dopamine receptors. Also, there is some evidence that psychotic phenomena like hearing voices are enhanced or even initiated by increased dopamine activity. This explains why many people who go on a cocaine or crystal binge end up getting paranoid, as these drugs release lots of dopamine in the brain.

Recent imaging evidence suggests that dopamine is involved in determining the salience of experiences so that an over-activity would lead to inappropriate salience attribution which could make people believe things are more relevant than they are, i.e. become paranoid.

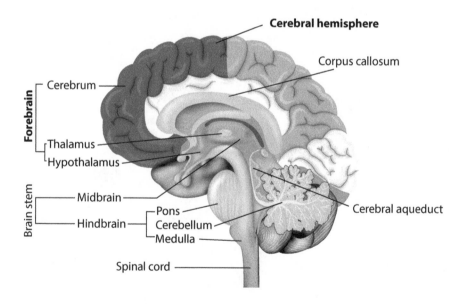

Figure 9: Brain regions and functions—Inside view of one hemisphere

CHAPTER 5

How the Cortex Works — Seeing is Believing

The example of paranoia I described at the end of *Chapter 4* is a good introduction to a fundamental concept of brain function, particularly that of the cortex. The brain is a biological machine and one of its major functions is to analyse and interpret information from the sense organs, linking them with relevant memories and creating hypotheses on which to act. As the pioneering German scientist Herman von Helmholtz (1821–1894) concluded over 150 years ago:

'The brain is an inference-making machine.'

This conclusion is probably surprising to many people who innocently assume that the eye sees the 'real' world and the ear 'hears' real sounds. On reflection this cannot be true since the eye is not a digital camera, nor the ear a recording disc. And if they were there would have to some other organ inside the brain that was acting as a viewer or listener (a miniature human or homunculus) and in that person's brain there would have to be the same homunculus again-and-again *ad infinitum*.

Sensations are 'perceived' by the brain as a result of analyses and reconstructions of the electrical impulses from the sense organs. The intensity, frequency and timing characteristics of these inputs define how the brain decides what the sensations from the real world actually are; these are called 'percepts.' The brain then directs movements appropriate to these percepts to benefit the person and also lays down memories of them if it seems likely they will be useful.

In some cases when the stimuli are too strong, memories are laid down despite their not being useful; the best example of this is in the case of post-traumatic stress disorder (PTSD) which we will discuss later in this chapter. In some cases, simple percepts can invoke enormous brain responses. A touch of silky cloth can invoke memories of an old lover with all the attendant emotions.

A famous example of a percept uncovering a whole plethora of memories and emotions was that of the French novelists Marcel Proust (1871–1922) who when tasting his favourite cake — the madeleine — in *Remembrance of Things Past* recounts how this percept allowed him to enter the complex and detailed world of his childhood. One survivor of the *Titanic* could never again listen to the music of 'The Tales of Hoffman.' This was the last piece of music she heard the orchestra playing before she was forced to evacuate the ship and it always brought back the memory, and associated terror, of being on the sinking ship.

Another PTSD sufferer who was a patient of mine escaped unhurt but very frightened from a burning railway carriage. They would re-experience the memory and fear of the episode whenever they smelt the unmistakable odour of train brakes heating up. Fear that this recollection would be reactivated by the smell of the brakes any time a train stopped meant they refused to travel by train again.

The mind's eye

The process of seeing is perhaps the most studied, and informative of just how complex this reality-detecting process in the brain is. When we view an object or scene, light from these enters both of our eyes through the lens of each. The refractive nature of each lens means the image projected onto the back of the retina is inverted and reversed. So, the first thing the brain has to do with any visual input is adapt to this reversal of side/side and top/bottom. The second is to merge the left and right eye inputs into a single stereoscopic image. These processes can be studied by giving volunteers prism glasses to wear that invert or 'left-right reverse' the world. At first the wearers find it impossible to walk or read because of the image inversion, but over a few days to weeks their brain adjusts to the point where things appear normal again. Of course, when the take the glasses off the visual inputs to each eye switch back to normal and the brain has to re-learn this former, but now new, orientation which it does over a few days.

The fact that the brain can do such sophisticated and rapid compensatory adjustments tells us that it has enormous flexibility or plasticity. It is a wonderful adaptive learning machine that gives humans such profound ability to adjust to different environments, which explains how we have achieved such evolutionary dominance. As Charles Darwin (1809–1892) explained, it is not the most powerful of the most specialised species that do best, it is those that are most adaptable to changing environmental pressures. Our brains are the best example of this adaptability in practice. The mechanisms underpinning this adaptability are not well understood but must involve alterations in neuronal and synaptic activity across wide areas of the brain. When (and if) these processes are ever decoded it seems likely that they will inform new ways of computing to create even better learning machines than the computers we have today.

Can these processes be encouraged, can flexibility of learning be enhanced? Again, this is conjectural at present but there is evidence that the neurotransmitter serotonin (*Chapter 2*) may play a role in allowing mental flexibility. Drug treatments that enhance serotonin, such as the SSRI antidepressants or the 5-HT2A receptor agonist psychedelic drugs can enhance brain flexibility in rodents and there is preliminary data for a similar effects in humans.

Getting back to how we see things, when light hits the back of the retina the light energy ('photons') then stimulate photo-receptors called rods and cones that contain modern derivatives of the bacterial rhodopsin introduced above. These photo-receptor cells transmute the light input into electrical outputs.

Rods are colour insensitive and largely detect location and movement, whereas cones are sensitive to one of three colours of light — red, green, or blue. Together they provide the exquisite colour sensitivity that humans possess. The electrical outputs of the retinal photo-receptor cells then pass through a neural net of multiple layers of neurons in the retina itself. These layers of neurons process the light intensity and colour information in a series of stages that transform them from being simple reflections of light intensity and colour into patterns that are multiplexed in both time and frequency domains. These complex, transformed images from the retina are then sent to the visual cortex in the brain via another relay station that performs further analysis on the way.

In the visual cortex these multiplexed inputs then begin a complex process of being reconstructed into what we call vision, in different places. The first processing occurs in primary visual cortex which puts the inputs back into a more topographic form, creating simple visual images of a few standard shapes. These constructs are then forwarded up to higher-level visual areas that pull them together into something more akin to a picture. But different areas mediate different aspects of the visual scene. One area is just responsible for analysing movement in the visual field, another content, another colour, and another place. Eventually when the inputs from these many different parts of the brain are integrated a complete 'image' or rather a perception of the visual scene is reconstructed.

But is it a true and faithful reconstruction? Of course not, to do such detailed real-time continuous reconstruction of visual inputs would be hugely complex and wasteful of resources. Most of what we 'see' is inferred by the brain so that only especially interesting or relevant parts of the visual space is dealt with in much detail, the rest is in effect 'made up.' The brain assumes it to be the same as it was in the previous few seconds. This can be beautifully demonstrated by the 'gorilla experiment.' Subjects are shown a short film in which a group of people are throwing a ball to each other in a game of catch. They are told their task is to count as accurately as they can how many times the ball is thrown. As the ball is moving around quickly across the screen counting each throw requires a considerable degree of attentional resources. So much so that most participants who take the exercise seriously do not see the man in a gorilla suit who walks through the film in the middle of the game! They see what they want and expect to see — the moving ball — and not what they don't expect (and don't want) to see — the man in a gorilla suit.

Another good example of how the visual brain works in a non-intuitive way is given by the illusion of backward rotation of spoked wheels of cars and carriages in movies and TV films. This apparent backward rotation is due to the fact that films and TV, unlike our visual system, do not provide a continuous measure of action, they cut it up into a number of frames — up to 650 a minute. Though we don't perceive this fragmentation, our brains do and see each frame as separate. So, when from one frame to the next the wheel spokes are in different positions the brain computes the shortest way the change in position of the spoke could have been made, which often would be by the wheel rotating backwards not forwards.

A related common experience that shows the brain makes estimates of change is that of feeling that the stationary train one is sitting in is moving when it's the train on the adjacent line that pulls out of the railway station. When sensory data can be interpreted in two ways the brain does what it is doing all the time, making the best decision for the person's survival, which in the case of the train seeming to move is to prepare the body for action rather than remaining static.

Seeing is still more complex. Once the key elements of a visual scene have been reconstructed so that novel shapes, colours and movements have been identified, then analysis on content and meaning take place in other brain regions. When we see a face, we don't just care if it's a face, we want to know whose face it is, what's their name, why are they here? Were we supposed to know that they would be here, when did we last see them, etc., etc? These questions involve digging into our enormous memory banks of faces and comparing the one in front of us with the stored data.

Often faces and people are identified in memory by where they are usually seen, which explains why we can walk past a friend in a new place such as an airport as our brain was not expecting an encounter them there. Then, once the face is identified as a friend, memory circuits orchestrated by the hippocampus are activated. These retrieve data on when and where the person was seen, who they are, how you met, what they do, how many children they have, what's their wife's name—sometimes is the woman with them their wife, or daughter? Or lover—in which case we rely on our frontal lobes to suppress our desire to ask!

The emotional memories are also explored and if these are positive then approach behaviour with a smile, a handshake or hugging may emerge. If our memory is negative then we may look away, frown and walk faster to avoid ourselves being recognised. We may even literally, as well as metaphorically, turn our back. These emotional responses are orchestrated from brain regions particularly the amygdala and insula. In fact, emotional recognition of threat is so important to the organism that it takes place first at a sub-conscious level. We can start running away from, or prepare to fight a threatening human or wild animal before realising exactly what it is. There is a natural and useful preparedness against threat that helps to keep us safe.

Here again we see how the brain's predictive inferential style of working comes into play. Everyone has experienced the feeling of being suddenly startled—we jump and look frightened. When in a threatening situation, e.g. in the classic horror movie scenario of walking through a graveyard on a dark night, we are already more aroused ('on edge') so any sudden noise or unexpected shape in the darkness can cause us to jump even more. Of course, this is often a vicious circle for as we become more fearful our visual system starts to assume the fear is reasonable so begins to see things as threatening that aren't—we develop illusions such as that a shadow is a ghost or an attacker.

For most people this is just embarrassing but such over-reactions can be damaging if they are activated inappropriately such as occurs in people with PTSD. They may react with fear and fight or flight reactions to innocuous noises or smells that remind them of their traumas. This can even happen when asleep and cases of Army veterans going on the attack are well-documented and on rare occasions can lead then fighting with and even killing partners in bed believing them to be the enemy.

The illusionary responding that anxiety or fear encourages is a major causative and perpetuating factor in some psychiatric conditions. People with anxiety states such as spider phobias often misinterpret cracks in walls or patterns in carpets as being spiders, so are always jumpy and on edge. PTSD is the result of being traumatised, but fear-induced inappropriate jumpy responding can lead to soldiers killing innocent bystanders. This leads to them becoming full of guilt that can result in depression and it also worsens the pre-existing PTSD.

Recall of times past? From seeing to remembering

At the top end of any visual input there is a decision to be made whether to remember the scene or not. Factors that make memory encoding more likely are intensity, novelty, pleasure and other emotional response and the importance of the scene. We can all remember emotional scenes such as an exam or driving test, and pleasurable ones such as our wedding or graduation days. Visiting beautiful or impressive sites such as the Taj Mahal or the Eiffel Tower are easily remembered not just because of their fame but also because we made the effort to get there that has been rewarded by their beauty and uniqueness.

In general, the more of the pro-memory factors engaged in any scene or other sensory input the stronger the memory.

Memories are laid down by a combination of increased glutamate activity and relative GABA inactivity, so allowing calcium influx into the neurons that are activated by the visual scene and the concomitant motives for memory storage. With fearful emotional visual memories activation of the brain's noradrenaline systems seem to play a crucial role by turning on brain emotion circuits in the same way it turns on the heart to beat faster. This knowledge has led to the development of drugs that block noradrenaline receptors. One of these is prazosin which is now being used as in the treatment of the unpleasant nightmares of PTSD, which are simply the trauma memories waking-up the patient from their sleep. Another new approach is to use a noradrenaline beta-receptor antagonist (a beta-blocker) to help desensitise trauma memories. The emotional elements of fear memories require noradrenaline acting through beta-receptors in the brain to be fully laid down. Beta-blockers can disrupt this process and so may be useful in therapy.

An important fact is that emotional memories are laid down despite the person not wanting them. They engage a subconscious circuit that has strong survival value. It ensures that all animals, not just we humans with conscious thoughts, can learn about the nature and occurrence of life-threatening risks and so protect ourselves against their occurring again in the future by avoidance or fighting. Such reflex fear responses can emerge without the person wanting them and in conditions like PTSD they occur despite the person trying to suppress them, which shows how powerful they can be.

In contrast to the fearful neurotransmitter noradrenaline, serotonin may have a necessary role in laying down positive emotional memories. We know that in depression people seem to be locked into a negative mind-set that encourages access of negative or 'bad' memories. In fact, in severe cases these memories may not even be true, they can be delusional. I have had depressed patients claim they have hurt or damaged others even though the victims confirm that this didn't occur. Also depressed people selectively see negative and bad things in their environment; their brains are set with a negative bias. When shown a neutral face they are more likely than non-depressed people to say it looks threatening or depressed. When SSRI antidepressants are given the first thing they do is to alter this bias so the depressed person's brain expresses a normal rather than distorted view of the world. This encourages them to act more normally, e.g. going out more, meeting old friends etc. These activities help them learn that the world is a nicer place than they had previously assumed. It may be this is the major mode of action of these drugs to lift mood, though in the long-term they also protect against recurrence of depression by promoting resilience through altering brain stress systems.

Where in the brain these internal hypotheses or inferences come from is a key question for brain science. We presume they are largely developed in the silent parts of the cortex. That's what these parts are thought to be doing, making sense of the multitude of sensory inputs by comparing them with the internal predictions, enacting relevant behaviour, monitoring the effects of this and adjusting the internal inferences accordingly. It's a massive task that no computer in the world could begin to emulate at present and is the result of years of experiential learning from birth to the teenage years (and even later for emotional and social learning).

Input is critical and may be very time dependent as has been shown by studies of visual and auditory development where critical time windows ('critical periods') are known. If someone is blind from birth due to a cataract in the lens of both eyes, then restoring site after the age of about five is unfortunately pointless as the visual system is fully-locked into its analytical processes by then. If normal visual input doesn't occur in childhood, then the visual system doesn't develop the underlying processes for seeing and never can. In practice in congenitally blind people much of the visual cortex becomes taken over to work for the auditory system which probably explains why blind people can have such superior hearing abilities; a lot more of their brain is given over to hearing.

Much more common is the effect of early hearing loss on speech development. Hearing deficits from ear infections are extremely prevalent in toddlers and, unlike blindness, may often not be known about by the parents. If left untreated such impairments of hearing can profoundly delay and limit speech development, so detecting hearing loss is a critical element in child care professionals such as health visitors, as simple surgical interventions such as grommets in the ear can restore adequate hearing and allow normal speech development.

What is remarkable is the precision with which the brain makes its inferences over decades of life. These allow us to function in a 'near-real' world that behaves largely according to our perceptions about its being real. However, when this predictive ability goes wrong significant problems emerge, such as schizophrenia and depression. As we have already seen in the case of Phineas Gage (*Chapter 3*), errors of high-level decision-making about social behaviours can emerge from damage to the frontal lobes. In later chapters we shall see how others occur in illness states and when under the influence of drugs.

Seeing things that aren't there

We can't leave a discussion of perception without mentioning the remarkable feature of the brain to make-up sensations and percepts if deprived of sensory input. This is seen most easily in the 'flotation tank' experiments where a person floats in absolute quiet in a dark room in water at body temperature so is denied any sensory input. Within a few minutes of sensory deprivation, the person begins to see lights and hear limited noises. Over time these hallucinations increase in scale and magnitude and can become like fully-fledged scenes such as experienced in dreaming. For many people this is very disturbing as they feel they are going mad; in fact, it is the nearest they may come to being psychotic. Some like the sense of escape from real world inputs and seek this out as a form of therapy.

Similar experiences are seen when people are accidentally deprived of alterations in sensory input, such as during a snowstorm or fog when images can develop as if they were outside, say of a car in the whiteness beyond. A classic case study showed this was common in a group of sailors who were in a race across the North Sea when becalmed in fog for over 24 hours. Most hallucinated badly, first seeing colours in the fog, then as time went on the hallucinations became more complex and realistic, they would 'see' other boats and people coming to rescue them out of the state of permanent whiteness. These experiences tell us that the experienced brain can generate any kind of sensory percept it likes from internal processes without input from the outside. When released from its normal role of having to deal with the continuous torrent of incoming sensory traffic the brain creates its own reality. This feature of brain function is almost certainly what generates dreams during sleep, which we discuss more in the next chapter. It also explains phenomena such as hallucinations and delusions, which are brain generated 'theories' of the world that are not anchored in reality as they are not linked to sensory inputs. However, they are 'real' to the person experiencing them, as they are perceived as being from the outside world. Even when it is obvious that they cannot be eternally generated, e.g. voices in a silent room, the brain will create a theory of how they are being generated, e.g. from a radio implanted in a tooth, or a transmitter in an ear. Such ideas are the basis of paranoid delusions that I describe in *Chapter 15*.

The autonomy of the brain to 'do its own thing' tells us that brain activity is not just a passive reactive process but that there are internal drives to action and activity. These come from a range of different neuronal types being 'pacemaker' cells that fire in a regular fashion because the ion pumps across their cell membranes slowly fade so that they periodically depolarise and fire-off action potentials that then activate many other neurons in the brain. These pacemaker neurons then re-polarise and the process begins again.

In this way the brain is always active, until when these cells stop firing when we die. The activity generating neurons are in the brain stem and are called the 'reticular activating system.' If their ascending projections are cut-off experimentally in animals, they go into a state of inactivity. This is replicated in humans following concussion and after rare immune attacks on the brain that produce what is known as the locked-in state. Basic functions such as breathing are maintained but higher functions stop, sometime to recover as the neural damage remits, or sometimes not: see *Chapter 7* for more on this state.

CHAPTER 6

Taking Control — From Urges to Self-discipline

Urges and drives are everyday experiences. We wake-up with a dry mouth and take a glass of water, then treat our overnight fast with food (breakfast). On the way to work we may see an attractive person and feel some kind of emotion, maybe lust or maybe a more cerebral pleasure. At work we may be bored but continue to perform out of fear of losing our job, or more likely because of the anticipated pleasures that the monthly salary cheque will bring. Coming home from work parents will feel the enormous warmth and affection of loving a child. Some children — at least when they are young — may even reciprocate the emotion! Then after another meal to deal with hunger, sleepiness begins to set in and we go to bed, sometimes for sex but always for sleep.

These drives for food, sleep, sex, etc. are all fundamental to mammalian life. They are hardwired into even the most primitive brain to ensure the life of the individual and the continuation of the species through reproduction. Drives involve a complex mixture of neuronal activity accompanied by hormonal changes driven from a brain region called the hypothalamus (see *Figures 8* and *9*).

Hormones are a form of neurotransmitter that spread through the blood rather than across synaptic gaps, so can influence many organ systems to prepare them for necessary bodily changes that fit with the brain's activities too. Many women experience this dual impact each month during their menstrual period when the changes in levels of the hormones progesterone and oestrogen alter the lining of the uterus and also change the brain to give headaches, altered emotions and sleep.

In some cases, the brain effects can be profound. For example, some forms of epilepsy only occur during the menstrual phase ('catamenial epilepsy'), probably because of the metabolism of progesterone in the brain leading to the production of the pro-convulsant chemical progesterone sulphate that is a weak blocker of GABA receptors. When progesterone levels are high then enough of the sulphate can be made to decrease GABA function and promote seizures.

Some cases of depression after childbirth (post-partum depression) are due to the profound fall of the hormone progesterone that occurs after the placenta is discharged. Progesterone levels are exceptionally high in pregnancy and fall precipitously after childbirth leading in some people to a withdrawal state that provokes depressed mood. A new medicine for the treatment of this form of depression has just been licensed, brexanolone. This is a synthetic version of the main metabolite of progesterone—allopregnanolone. This hormone promotes GABA function in the brain and is responsible for the tranquillity and memory impairments that are commonly reported by pregnant women (a state my wife and mother of our four children called dementia gravidarum). Brexanolone is a synthetic version of allopregnanolone that is given intravenously for 60 hours in women with post-partum depression to rectify the hormone imbalance that causes the mood drop. Perhaps surprisingly, chemically related GABA hormone drugs that can be taken orally also seem to work in other forms of depression and may reach the market in due course.

In other species we know that menstrual hormone changes are associated with profound remodelling of parts of the nervous system that prepare the animal for sex and then parenthood. For example, when a female cat is in heat there is a massive increase in the number of synapses in that part of the spinal cord that is responsible for copulation. The cat also exudes pheromones (air-borne hormones) that attract males for mating. Although we can't say for sure that menstrual hormone changes affect female human nervous systems in exactly the same way it seems likely that similar neuronal alterations do occur. Certainly, there is evidence of altered activity of human female pheromones during the menstrual cycle, and these seem to entrain groups of women who live in the same house to synchronise their menstrual cycles.

Other hormones that change behaviour in predictable ways are testosterone and oxytocin. As males enter puberty testosterone levels rise. This leads to the classic behaviours of this phase of life—a sudden development of interest in those who attract us sexually, new grooming behaviour to make oneself acceptable to such people, and repetitive thinking about sex. Usually there is an increase in muscle mass along with a deepening of the voice associated with brain changes that increase aggression. All these changes have significant evolutionary value as they are used to assist in obtaining and protecting female mates and subsequent children. Today such testosterone-fuelled aggression is often a problem unless deflected into warfare or more humane proxies for fighting such as contact sports.

Oxytocin is the hormone that mothers secrete when breast feeding their babies. When the baby suckles, nerves from the breast induce the release of oxytocin from the pituitary gland at the base of the brain and into the blood. This circulating oxytocin helps the let-down of milk and its replenishment. But the suckling process also releases oxytocin in certain parts of the brain which bonds the mother to the baby, one of several reasons breast-feeding is preferred to bottle feeding.

Oxytocin is also released during orgasm and is thought to aid bonding between partners in the post-coital phase. As MDMA (ecstasy) also releases oxytocin this may account for this drug's rather unique ability to enhance loving feelings and empathy between people (so called 'entactogenic' effects). For these reasons, many groups have tried to encourage loving or positive social behaviour — or at least reduce aggression — by giving oxytocin — for example in people with autism.

Despite many positive claims (and probably as many if not more unpublished negative results) the jury is still out on whether oxytocin is a potential treatment or not. One reason is that it is still not known if oxytocin given into the blood or as a spray into the nose, actually gets into the brain. Another issue is that the effects of oxytocin are gender specific. While it may reduce some forms of aggression in men it can increase them in women of childbearing age, presumably to help them to fight off threats to their children.

Hormone production and release are controlled from an evolutionary old part of the brain called the hypothalamus. This links the brain to the pituitary gland from which many hormones are released into the blood. The hypothalamus and pituitary also produce and secrete other types of hormones that travel to glands such as the adrenal and testes/ovaries where they stimulate the production and release of large quantities of other hormones such as cortisol, testosterone, and oestrogens. The hypothalamus also contains groups of neurons called nuclei that not only each regulate particular hormones, but also orchestrate relevant behavioural responses that support the hormonal effects and often precede them. Experimental stimulation of these nuclei can lead to a range of primary behaviours such as eating, drinking, fear and fighting. Other nuclei in the hypothalamus regulate sex and the sleep-wake cycle.

The combined actions of these nuclei in the hypothalamus therefore provide the lowest level of a fully-integrated brain where basic life support functions are driven and coordinated. It tells us when to eat drink and sleep, and when to have sex and reproduce. In Freudian terms it represents the id, the centre for 'primitive' drives that are biologically necessary, but that need to be curbed and controlled for normal or at least desirable human society to flourish.

The constraints on the hypothalamus are provided by descending inputs from higher up in the more evolutionary recent parts of the brain, particularly the cortex. These regions have developed in most mammals to control—or perhaps better—direct the drives and urges that come from the hypothalamus. A great deal of child rearing and later education is directed at teaching the growing cortex to control these urges and so the child learns to behave more and more like an adult. It can be taught to wait to start eating until the adults are ready and only to eat food on its plate. It can be taught to pee and poo in a loo rather than on the floor, and as a teenager to control sexual urges and express them in private.

As we have seen with the example of Phineas Gage (*Chapter 3*) a major role of the frontal lobe is to control urges and so regulate behaviour. Gage's behaviour changed for the worse as a result of damaging this part of his brain. We see similar deficits in social behaviour and urge control in people with dementia, especially in those in which the frontal lobes are damaged early. Such patients can become very disinhibited—taking food from other peoples' plates and being violent and aggressive when asked to desist!

One way to view the function this frontal part of the cortex is in terms of the Freudian concepts of ego and super-ego, the former being those thoughts and feelings that represent the true 'us' and the latter those behaviours and ambitions that we—or more usually our parents and teachers—want us to be. The ego can be to some extent identified as a circuit in the cortex called the default mode network (DMN). This circuit is formed from integrated activity from the frontal lobe and a region in the middle of the back of the brain called the posterior cingulate cortex. When a person is quietly reflecting on their life, their plans and thwarted ambitions, the default mode network is highly active. In depressive states with ruminations of guilt and failure it can become overactive and 'lock' the person into a negative mind-set (see *Chapter 13*).

The super-ego is less easy to locate but could be construed as being located partly in the DMN and in other more lateral frontal cortical regions. These apply descending controls over the ego and id in an attempt to try to regulate them both. This top-down kind of moral control of behaviour may fail and unwelcome disruptive urges and drives can then dominate a person's behaviour. This breakdown can be permanent, e.g. caused by brain damage as with Phineas Gage, or transient, as with intoxication with alcohol and cocaine when they can lead to violent or sexually-disinhibited behaviours. In other people the super-ego can develop excessively and dominate and distort normal behaviour so that states of worry and other forms of neurosis develop. It can also suppress many, if not all, of the basic drives so, for example in monks and nuns sexual desires are totally suppressed and even eating and drinking subject to extreme regulation.

Other examples of top-down control from the cortex overriding more primitive self-protection drives are seen in war. Here training and group dynamics plus a deep commitment to 'the cause' leads to military personnel overcoming fear and escape drives and fight even though they know they are very likely to die (e.g. the Somme offensive in World War I) or even to deliberately kill themselves along with the enemy (e.g. Japanese kamikaze pilots in World War II). These individuals 'died for the glory and security of their State'; modern Islamic suicide bombers do so, usually in the belief they will have a special place in Heaven.

The power of the cortex to override normal emotional reactions is seen frequently in other aspects of life. A frightening example was the Holocaust where the extermination of Jews, gypsies, the mentally-ill and others was conducted by 'normal' German soldiers (as documented in the book *Ordinary Men* by Christopher Browning: see *Selected Bibliography*), often in opposition to their true beliefs and ethical principles. Human beings did this because they came to believe that obeying orders from the Third Reich was more important than acting on the empathy they had for the humans they were murdering.

Normally these elements of brain action develop in a balanced way and remain in equilibrium unless some brain insult such as alcohol destabilises this. However, in some cases neural development doesn't occur in equilibrium and then one or other levels can dominate. A common example of this is attention deficit hyperactivity disorder (ADHD), a condition where children (and some adults) are always 'on the go,' with short attention spans, an inability to sit still and concentrate, and poor sleep. This disorder can severely damage their schooling and often leads to them failing at school and then dropping-out into a life of petty crime and eventually ending up in prison (up to 25% of UK prisoners are thought to have ADHD: see Susan Young et al in the *Selected Bibliography*).

The brain mechanisms of ADHD seem to be a failure of the frontal lobes to control motor drives emerging from the basal ganglia and hypothalamus. This failure is partly because of delayed maturation of the frontal lobes, as they are the last part of the brain to become fully functional. When they do mature enough to control the urge to move and explore, from the teenage years onwards, then ADHD begins to remit. Sadly, this doesn't occur in everyone and up to 15 per cent of childhood cases of ADHD persist well into adulthood. The frontal lobes can be helped to work more efficiently by medications such as methylphenidate (Ritalin) that augment dopamine and noradrenaline function in this region and so improve attention and concentration.

The fact that drugs like methylphenidate calm hyperactive patients with ADHD, rather than activate them like they do in the majority of people, tells us that ADHD is definitely a brain disorder and not just some form of social labelling. Perhaps the most vivid demonstration of this fundamental difference in brain function comes from the response to stimulants taken at night; many ADHD patients find that these drugs help them sleep rather than keep them awake! Some cocaine users find that this stimulant encourages them to sit down and read a book for the first time rather than go partying with their mates, proof again that dopamine helps their attention, and their brain is organized differently from that of other people.

Another example of a failure of top-down super-ego control is mania (see *Chapters 6* and *15*). Here the cortex is functioning normally, but the drives become so powerful that they override it leading to the breakthrough of excessive sexual activity, often with altered gender and person preference, lessened sleep and a sense of energy that can border on omnipotence. The sleep deficit then aggravates the illness and can lead to an upward spiral of manic mood that may culminate in delusions of grandeur, dangerously disinhibited behaviour and, if untreated, death.

The opposite side of the urge-control system is autism. Here the top-down control is thought to be excessive and dominate basic drives. This leads to high levels of anxiety, particularly in social situations, with avoidance of eye-contact, introspection and self-centred behaviours such as rocking and skin picking that seem to serve an anxiety-reducing function. So far, we have made disappointing progress in finding treatments for autism. One new approach is to try oxytocin to improve social bonding, though with the caveats mentioned above. Another is to use the empathogenic and anxiolytic properties of MDMA to reduce social anxiety, and a pilot trial of this is ongoing in the USA.

Eating disorders can also be seen as a malfunction of the usual balance between the hypothalamic drive to eat and the cortical regulation of this. In many people excess intake of food leads to obesity, which largely reflects the easy cheap access to high calorie and high fat foods in the modern diet. Our brains' relationship to food is still in the mode they were when we were hunter-gatherers evolving in Africa. Food was hard to come by, so any and all food was a precious resource that had to be consumed in case it was the last for a long time. In some rare cases such as the Prader-Willi syndrome this drive for food is greatly exaggerated (or more accurately fails to satiate). This failure to control the urge to eat means that if allowed unlimited access to food such patients consume vastly more than the average person, maybe three-to-five times as much, which means that before they reach their teenage years they are severely overweight.

Patients with bulimia also binge on food, usually in an attempt to compensate for psychological distress. This can lead to weight gain unless they also learn how to vomit after they gorge, which prevents the excess calorie intake, but the regurgitated acid can damage their teeth and produce major disturbances of blood chemistry.

The obverse of bulimia is anorexia (nervosa), a condition where there is excessive cortical suppression of the desire to eat that leads to severe malnourishment and has a death rate of 15 per cent, similar to that of other major psychiatric disorders such as addiction, major depression and schizophrenia. Anorexia is, par-excellence, a disorder of the super-ego driving the person to try to achieve perfection of shape and physiology. This ideal is conceived as a fashionably skinny, ageless (in fact perpetually pre-reproductive age) woman and is obtained by an unrelenting will to deny the desire and need to eat. The food restriction and weight loss then leads to amenorrhoea which further perpetuates the pre-pubertal image by limiting breast growth.

CHAPTER 7

Thinking, Feeling and Consciousness

One of the great challenges to science is the understanding of consciousness. A challenge almost as great is how to define it? Consciousness is something we all understand at an intuitive level, it's the awareness we have of being awake and doing things, of noticing how we are behaving, what we are thinking about, etc. Some philosophers have suggested that consciousness is the central element of being human, and though it seems likely that other species have some forms of self-awareness this is unlikely to be as sophisticated as ours because of the quite special human aptitude of language.

Consciousness seems to be an 'emergent' property of the brain; something that only can occur or emerge once the basic structure and neuronal pathways of the brain have been put into place and then fine-tuned by use and experience. Because it seems to relate to brain size and complexity it is possible that other large-brained mammals such as dogs, elephants and dolphins have some form of consciousness — they certainly have volition and emotions and forms of social communication, plus in some cases self-awareness. As their brains have evolved to their current large size independently of ours, this suggests an interesting concept — at some point as brain size and complexity increases, consciousness emerges. The brains of these species and ours all diverged from common ancestors with very small brains, so the expansion of the size of their brains is independently driven though with essentially the same basic structure and organization as ours. There may also have been independent evolution of self-awareness as it has been reported in the crow species of birds whose evolutionary path diverged from ours well before the emergence of mammals.

The implications of this are that brains evolve and grow larger and more sophisticated in different species and that, at some point, the increased brain size and structure adds some extra component—such as self-awareness—to its basic abilities. This can be construed as forms of consciousness. Whether these other large-brained creatures can experience other human consciousness phenomena such as imagination or religious belief is unknowable since they don't have language. But dogs have been shown in experimental studies to have moral values and dolphins have been observed seeking out drug-induced altered states by sucking toxins out of puffer fish. I know that many dog-owners feel their pets have meaningful engagement with them emotionally and some dogs can also develop false beliefs as indicated by superstitious-like behaviours. Films like the American CNN documentary 'Blackfish' (2013) by Gabriella Cowperthwaite and her co-directors have suggested that dolphins and killer whales may also have some kind of moral intentionality.

The language of consciousness

There can be little argument with the premise that the evolved modification of the human brain that allowed language to develop was the most important one in the history of life after that of the evolution of DNA/RNA. Remarkably these two processes are unique in that they both work because they use abstract symbolic constructs to direct activity. The language of DNA is one where a small number of 'words' are built up of three letters, each letter being a small chemical (nucleotide). Then via RNA these triplets code for the amino-acid sequence in proteins. Francis Collins the Head of the Human Genome Project called this 'The language of God.'

Human language is considerably more complex and sophisticated. Building blocks of different sounds lead to the spoken language and symbolic visual images to the written word. Language is encoded in a special way in the brain—it is lateralised. In right-handed people language is located on the left side of the brain. This explains why strokes that impair movements of the right side of the body are strongly associated with loss of language (aphasia), for the left cerebral hemisphere controls the right side of the body. In about half of left-handed people language is in the right hemisphere and in the other half it is on the left—a phenomenon called mixed hemispheric dominance. One explanation of the predominance of right-handedness in humans is that language laterality came first, and this directed motor lateralisation.

The fact that mastery of the extreme complexity of language(s) can be gained by young children with seemingly no effort tells us the development of language ability is clearly something inherent in the brain. Also, although fluent spoken language requires the ability to hear, the underlying rules of language don't. Congenitally deaf people are perfectly capable of reading and writing even if their hearing of speech is non-existent and their speech production is, usually, very poor or absent altogether. On the other hand, there are some individuals, most commonly men, who have specific deficits in reading ability, and this has a strong genetic basis. Presumably, these genes encode for processes that help the organization of the reading language centres of the brain. It seems likely that future research into exactly what they do will unlock more of the marvellous mechanisms of language.

The ability of humankind to download its knowledge and ideas into the spoken and then the written word has been the critical factor in the growth of our species to dominate all others and the world itself. Knowledge truly is power. And now the internet gives us all access to almost everything that has ever been written and known, so we as a species have a truly remarkable ability to empower ourselves. But though language is a hugely flexible and expandable process it also can constrain the way we address issues and problems. To some extent we think as language tells us to think. Scientific ideas are largely determined by the language in which they are expounded.

In the same way as Ludwig Wittgenstein (1889–1951) pointed out that philosophy is in essence a question of language and meaning, the way we consider the question of consciousness is structured by the nature of the language we use. But as physics was revolutionised by the concepts of relativity and quantum theory, our understanding of consciousness might be similarly revolutionised once we gain other insights and ways of understanding integrated brain function.

Staying awake — and alive!

Language gives us the ability to share and discuss the experiences of consciousness. But there is more to consciousness than the word. Consciousness almost certainly does not originate from just the language system in the brain. Lesions (damage) to different cortical regions can produce very different subjective as well as objective effects on brain function. If the frontal lobes are damaged, then judgement and planning are affected. If the parietal (lateral) lobes become impaired, then geographical location and route planning are disrupted (as commonly seen in Alzheimer's disease which starts in these regions and often leads to people with this condition getting lost). These observations confirm what we know of more obvious sensory and motor functions, they have specific localisations in the brain.

One remarkable brain state that is thankfully rare is that of 'locked-in syndrome.' Here individuals are frozen — as if in a coma — but are fully-aware of their environment. They can't move or speak but can hear see and feel. This originates from damage to an area in the brain stem — that part between the brain and spinal cord — where the dopamine and noradrenaline neuronal cell bodies are located. Damage here can be caused by head injury, a local stroke or by an immune attack on the neurons such as in Von Economo's disease, a rare adverse effect of the Spanish Flu epidemic in the early-1900s. Locked-in states with reduced external consciousness can be misdiagnosed as terminal brain coma unless careful attempts are made to ensure that the brain is still working. The work of Adrian Owens and colleagues using fMRI imaging with these patients has shown they are capable of complex thought and so quite conscious. When they are in the fMRI-scanner he asks the patients to imagine playing tennis and if they are conscious when doing so this activates their brain motor planning areas in a consistent fashion.

In contrast extreme sedation, e.g. from poisoning with alcohol or other sedatives or intentionally produced in anaesthesia comes from switching-off another part of the lower brain — the thalamus (*Figure 8*). This region converts the outputs of brain stem arousal-producing centres into an organized activation of the cortex that allows all its parts to do their own thing as well as interact with each other. Experimental studies of anaesthesia have shown that as the level of arousal drops activity in the neuronal circuits from thalamus to cortex reduce until, when deep coma is produced, they are silent.

Because the correct level of arousal is so important to the organism there are multiple neurotransmitter systems that each provide arousal to the cortex. This 'belt and braces' approach makes evolutionary sense—you don't want to suddenly fall asleep in a position where you might be vulnerable. But sometimes medical conditions can make this happen, and the most well-known of these is narcolepsy. This is a medical syndrome where the person gets sudden attacks of severe and irresistible sleepiness during the daytime. We have all experienced this kind of sleepy feelings when we are extremely tired or jet lagged but in patients with narcolepsy they happen on a regular basis even after a good night's sleep. These sleep attacks are often associated with a loss of muscle tone, so the patient falls forward over their desk or into a meal on the table, often with messy consequences. These episodes are called 'cataplectic' attacks, as the medical term for the sudden loss of muscle tone is cataplexy.

Other animals can experience similar attacks and much of the basic research work on this disorder was conducted in Stanford University, California, USA with a colony of Pointer dogs that could have the attacks provoked simply by offering them food! The prospect of eating excited them so much that they then collapsed, just like some humans with narcolepsy do when laughing or otherwise excited.

Until recently narcolepsy was a mysterious condition that sometimes occurred in young people after a viral infection but more commonly was seen in middle-aged men. For decades we have been treating it with stimulant drugs such as amphetamine (speed) to keep them awake and with SSRIs to reduce the cataplexy. One of the great achievements of molecular biology and receptor cloning in medicine has been the elucidation of the underlying neurobiology of this disorder. Groups in the USA and Japan working on the brain mechanisms of sleep and eating discovered a peptide neurotransmitter that affected these processes, but being unaware of each other's research, one group called it orexin (appetite suppressing hormone) and the other hypocretin. Once the peptide was identified it was possible to clone the receptor and gene and then produce mice in which either the receptor or the production of the hormone was eliminated—so called 'KO mice.' These showed sudden attacks of sleepiness suggesting orexin was a wake-producing hormone. Subsequently this was proved when spinal tap studies in humans with narcolepsy found very low levels of orexin in their cerebrospinal fluid. This has now become a diagnostic test for the disorder.

Why do humans with narcolepsy have low levels of orexin? It seems that this is a degenerative disorder, similar to Parkinson's disease. Probably the orexin cells die either from some internal problem of metabolism or from immune attacks, with the latter the most likely for the early onset cases.

There is growing evidence that very many disorders from ulcerative colitis to multiple sclerosis are due to the body's immune system attacking specific proteins on different organs (so called autoimmune disorders). The brain is less affected because it is to some extent protected by a membrane called the blood-brain-barrier that keeps blood borne toxins (and antibodies) out, but more and more neurologic and psychiatric conditions are becoming revealed as auto-immune in causation though the target protein (antigen) is not identified for all. For example, the common throat infection in children caused by streptococcus bacteria can lead to strange movements of the limbs colloquially known for several hundreds of years as Sydenham's Chorea. This is due to antibodies against the bacterium cross-reacting with a neuronal group in the dopamine rich areas of the brain that control movement—the basal ganglia. The movements though disturbing to parents and child usually stop as the infection comes under control but can return when another infection occurs. In some of these children, obsessive behaviours also develop. Other brain syndromes—such as some forms of epilepsy and even psychosis—are now known to be due to such brain targeted autoimmune attacks. Collectively these immune-brain disorders of children are known as PANDAS syndrome (Paediatric Autoimmune Neuropsychiatric Disorder Associated with Streptococci).

As well as giving us new insights into brain dysfunction and the mechanisms of some disorders, diagnosis of autoimmune brain disorders offers new approaches to treatment. The simplest is to give antibiotics every time an infection seems to be brewing to stop the bacteria multiplying. Once the syndromes have set in, then anti-inflammatory drugs may help though not much. The most effective treatment is a form of blood dialysis called plasmapheresis where the patient's blood is passed through an extra-corporeal machine (a bit like a kidney dialysis machine) that strips antibodies out of the plasma before the blood is returned to the patient. This is an expensive treatment that is not widely available but does prove the principle of immune attack on the brain being the cause of the problem.

The discovery from narcolepsy that sleep is due to a failure of orexin to be produced or — in some cases deficits in orexin receptor function — gave us a new treatment target for insomnia. If orexin keeps you awake then blocking its actions should put people to sleep, or at least keep them asleep.

Several pharmaceutical companies developed orexin receptor antagonist drugs and the one produced by Merck & Co (BELSOMRA® or suvorexant) has recently been approved as a treatment for insomnia in the USA. It helps prevent arousal-induced awakenings leading on to a full-blown waking episode. So, it improves the continuity of sleep that in turn results in the subjective sense of a better night's sleep.

Such scientific based treatment innovations are however rare in psychiatry with perhaps the only other example being in Alzheimer's disease. Here the discovery of a major loss of the critical memory neurotransmitter acetylcholine led to drugs such as donepezil and galantamine that help restore its activity with a positive impact on memory functions in some patients.

CHAPTER 8

The Emotional Brain

Emotions are one of the key features of all our lives. We laugh and cry, get angry and sad, worried and fearful. They have powerful effects on behaviour and in evolutionary terms have developed for just this reason, to direct behaviours for animal—and human—survival. They also are old in evolutionary terms in that we see similar behaviours in all mammals and in some birds.

Emotions start early in life—from the day we or born when affiliative loving interactions between mother and child are a vital aspect of bonding. These interactions are driven initially in the baby by the smell, touch and taste of breast milk and by all the senses plus the hormones, oxytocin and prolactin, in the mother. Touching stroking and cuddling may well release serotonin in the touch-responsive emotional circuit described in the section on serotonin in *Chapter 2*, perhaps helping to lay down positive mood traits that could persist into later life. Soon the baby also develops the ability to see the mother's smile and hear her voice. A failure to bond and be given sufficient sensory input can lead to delayed and stunted brain growth as was seen in the deprived children rescued from the Romanian orphanages.

The brain circuits of love are not well explored for although rodents and other mammals show tender parenting for a few days this soon diminishes as the babies gain autonomy much faster than the human baby. We suppose that they are part of the limbic system which is a sub-cortical network, parts of which are the hippocampus and amygdala. Other parts include the hypothalamus, which controls hormone release and many fundamental appetitive and sleep behaviours, plus parts of the cortex especially the insula and anterior cingulate cortex. This circuit is preserved in all mammals and may be selected for in domestic dogs and cats which often show intense affiliation with their owners, and each other. For dogs social bonding is critical to the organization and functioning of the pack which is why they bond so well with humans too.

The converse of affiliative emotions are the negative ones of fear, anxiety and depression. They also emerge from the limbic system though with significant cortical elements also. A key node in regulating negative emotions are the two amygdalae, buried deep inside each temporal lobe. These provide a sub-consciousness detection system for threat stimuli, detecting threats from human facial expression before the cortex can. The amygdala is tightly connected to lower brain regions that mediate the range of fear and escape responses as well as producing warning signals to other humans such as facial expressions of fear or terror and shrieks or gasps of alarm. Just as we saw in *Chapter 4* that for optimal survival the sensory motor system needs to respond to pain without thinking so the amygdala provides responses much faster than those derived from the cortex to deal with social cues and external threats.

The amygdala doesn't just deal with threats because it also seems to be responsive to positive facial expressions as well as to negative ones, though to a lesser extent. This amygdala functioning can be seen as a thermostat for emotional state. In people with depression the amygdala shows enhanced responses to fearful faces and reduced responses to happy ones, and antidepressant drugs, particularly the SSRIs remedy this bias towards negative facial inputs.

The work of Cath Harmer and Phil Cowen in Oxford has shown that antidepressant drugs quite rapidly attenuate this state of exaggerated responding to negative stimuli in the amygdalae. Because the full antidepressant drug response takes weeks to be fully apparent, they suggest that this resetting of the amygdala sensitivity may be the key to their action. Once people no longer have the reflex avoidance responses from the super-sensitive amygdala they can better engage with the world and other people. When they do this, they discover that the world is not as threatening and unpleasant a place as their depressed amygdala told them it was. Also, they obtain positive feedback on themselves. Together these two sets of experiences slowly lift their depression.

CHAPTER 9

Getting Inside the Head — Surgery to Imaging Techniques

The brain is quite difficult to study, because it is well-protected by a thick bony capsule called the skull. This is vital to insulate the very soft, nervous tissue from harm and keep the brain in correct alignment with the spinal cord, but it means that we can't directly explore brain function except when the bone has been removed as for instance in cases of brain surgery. This approach has been and continues to be a fruitful one but is still limited — you can't ask a health volunteer to have a hole cut in their skull just for scientific research!

Of course we can take advantage of illnesses and accidents to explore the relationship between changes in brain function before death and anatomical alterations seen at post-mortem, and this has been a most fruitful approach to understanding which bits of the brain do what — compare the case of Phineas Gage (*Chapter 3*) and the loss of his frontal lobe. A lot of data was collected after warfare where bullets and shrapnel would take out chunks of the brain and result in altered function such as the loss of sight if the visual region was damaged or paralysis of a limb if the motor cortex was injured. Also, post-mortem studies have revealed that dementias, e.g. Alzheimer's disease are associated with a great shrinkage of brain tissue and some memory deficits such as those produced by alcohol addiction.

Before the modern period of neurology, post-mortem studies were simply descriptive of the shape and structure of the brain as in Leonardo da Vinci's beautiful drawings. Strangely though at that time it was thought that key processes of the brain were not the soft tissue, but the fluid contained within it in the so-called brain ventricles!

This concept was a direct continuation of the ideas of the Ancient Greeks who believed that bodily processes and health were mediated by the four 'humors': black bile, yellow bile, blood and phlegm. An excess of black bile (*melaina chole*) was believed to lead to depression, hence the term we still sometimes use today for severe depression, melancholia. The ventricles of the brain were believed to be the store of these humors. At that time, the heart was seen as the dominant organ of human existence being considered the seat of the soul, rather than the pump of the blood we know it to be today.

This rather simplistic concept of brain function was gradually overturned by more systematic research by leading clinicians and brain researchers in the 18th and 19th centuries. From observations and brain dissections made post-mortem in people who had suffered brain damage from strokes, tumours or warfare they began to identify the sites of some more explicit brain functions such as movement and speech. The discrete differentiation of speech processes was a major breakthrough with Carl Wernicke (1848–1905) discovering the region of the brain that was required for the understanding of speech and Paul Broca (1824–1880) discovering that spoken language was produced from a different area. Along with this came the developments that emerged from the invention of the microscope which allowed the identification of the building blocks of the brain, the neurons. Together these were the foundation of modern brain science.

Still, getting to discover what actually goes on in the brain was impossible, and breakthroughs came slowly. The development of neurosurgery was utilised by pioneer neuroscientists such as Roger Sperry (1913–1994) to examine the activities of different brain regions. For example, once inside the skull it was possible to see what happened if a part of the brain was stimulated by touch or electrical stimuli. This approach found that different parts of the brain—later called the motor (movement) cortex—were responsible for different limb movements. This cortical region was shown to have a map of the body built within it. This map was not a true proportional representation of the body, though, because it became clear that much more of the cortex was involved in regulating activity of body parts that had complex movement abilities, e.g. the hand—whereas the amount of cortex involved in parts with more limited movements, e.g. the legs was much less. This means that the more complex the activity the more of the cortex is required to control it.

Stimulation of other brain regions produced very different effects. In some regions, sensations would be elicited — that of touch from the sensory cortex and simple visual images from the visual cortex. Other regions could lead to feelings of warmth or of anxiety and sometimes of *deja-vu* (the sense of having seen or experienced something before). However not all regions of the brain appeared to respond to stimulation and what they did remained a mystery that was only really revealed by the development of brain imaging methods. These regions were called silent cortex, in contrast to those that were responsive — the so-called eloquent cortex as when stimulated they 'spoke back.'

Neurosurgery wasn't just limited to the cortex, sometimes it went deeper to remove tumours and to remove dead tissue that was causing fits in epilepsy, the epileptic foci. These were often in the hippocampus and, in a few patients, there were foci on both sides of the brain so both were removed.

This operation often dramatically reduced the number of seizures, but a new and unexpected problem emerged — they lost the ability to store new memories though could still access ones that had been laid down previously. The experience of these patients proved that the hippocampus was the critical part of memory formation.

The memory loss produced by bilateral hippocampal surgery was quite similar to that described a century before in alcoholics by the Russian neurologist Sergei Korsakoff (1854–1900). His patients also could not lay down new memories but could remember the past. Post-mortem studies revealed that in alcoholic amnesia there was localised destruction of two small regions of the brain called the mammillary bodies. We now know that memory formation requires a functioning circuit that comprises the hippocampi, mammillary bodies and some other sub-cortical brain regions though the content of the memories themselves are probably stored in different parts of the cortex.

There are limits to how much we can understand from surgical and other invasive approaches, so researchers have for several centuries sought for non-invasive ways to measure what's going on in the brain. In the 1800s, phrenology was popular; it was believed that by feeling the shape of the skull inferences could be made about underlying brain capacity and psychological functioning. Although this is now seen as a ridiculous approach it was still popular in non-scientific circles well into the last century. The first scientific breakthrough in using external machinery to measure changes in brain activity came in the 1920s with the development of sensitive electrical amplifiers that allowed the measurement of electrical activity emerging from the brain. This technique is called EEG or electro-encephalography and is widely used to help diagnose epilepsy and to measure the different sleep stages. Electrodes are placed over the head and the changes in electrical potential across the different electrodes are measured and these are colloquially called 'brain waves.' The use of EEG revealed a range of different electrical frequencies from the brain that change during alertness and sleep. It is also used to detect brain responses to sensory stimuli, and even intentions, using a technique called evoked response potential (ERP) measurement.

One drawback of EEG it that it suffers from artefacts due to the electrical activity of the muscles attached to the skull and this can make analyses, particularly in the higher frequency ranges, inaccurate or even impossible. This issue can be to some extent overcome using a more modern technique called magneto-encephalography (MEG) that uses highly sensitive magnetic sensors called SQIDS (superconducting quantum interference devices) to measures the changes in magnetic fields that the underlying changes in electrical activity inevitably produce. MEG has been used to produce extremely clear images of the effects of different drugs on brain function, in effect 'fingerprinting' them.

Neither EEG or MEG can measure changes in deep brain structures, they largely give an indication of what's going on in the cortex. To look deep into the brain we need techniques that measure transmission throughout the brain and these are either magnetic (MRI) or radio-activity (PET or SPECT) based. MRI and PET allow us to plot the circuits that are active during performing tasks such as trying to remember. With modern high-field fMRI (functional magnetic resonance imaging) it is possible to plot in real time the brain regions activated in this process from seeing the to-be-remembered object through to depositing the memory into different parts of the brain via the hippocampus. So how do these machines work?

MRI and PET work in very different ways and each has its advantages and disadvantages. Both can be used to measure brain activity so as to identify the brain regions involved in any particular function. The MRI technique called functional or fMRI is now the most used because of its being a lot cheaper than PET, and it does not use radioactivity and gives better time-resolution. However PET was the first technique to allow us to measure brain action and many of the pioneering studies were done using radioactive water or radioactive glucose that are injected intravenously, then travel to the brain from where the radioactivity breaks down and emits gamma rays. With both techniques the head is placed in a large cylinder (the camera or scanner) that contains the detecting devices. In PET the camera really is a sort of camera as it detects the radioactivity from the tracer that is injected using photomultiplier crystals. It can be used to measure radioactivity from any molecular source injected and the special unique ability of PET is to allow us to measure receptors in the human brain not just metabolic activity. Moreover for a few neurotransmitters, with dopamine being the best example, PET allows us to estimate the release of a neurotransmitter in specific brain areas.

With fMRI the physics is quite different, the scanner is a hugely powerful circular magnet thousands of times stronger than the earth's magnetic field. This magnetises some molecules in the brain and blood (such as water and haemoglobin), so they all align with the magnetic field. Then special frequency radio waves are pulsed across the head and these for a short time (milliseconds) change the alignment of many of the magnetised molecules. When the radio wave pulse is switched-off they then relax back into their previous alignment and, as they do this, they give out their own radio signals that can be detected outside the skull. Then using Nobel Prize-winning mathematics these emitted radio signals are computed into measures of brain structure and function.

The water molecule signal is used to measure structure and the haemoglobin signal can measure brain blood flow and by proxy brain activity by a technique called blood oxygen level dependence or BOLD. This makes clever use of the fact that when haemoglobin loses oxygen its magnetic properties become much more pronounced so can be used to give a good signal in the scanner. Under most circumstances the more active a region of the brain is, the more blood flow goes to it. This means the fMRI signal from more active regions is different from that in less active ones and so changes in activity over seconds can be imaged. For example, moving one's right thumb will (in right-handed people) increase activity and blood flow in the left motor cortex, something so clearly seen on the fMRI scanner it can be used to calibrate it.

What have these two imaging techniques told us that we didn't know from post-mortem and surgical studies? Well PET has shown that there are deficits in neurotransmitters such as GABA in disorders where post-mortem studies are almost non-existent, e.g. anxiety disorders. It has also extended our knowledge of the pathology of depression and schizophrenia suggesting deficits of 5-HT receptors in depression and increased dopamine function in schizophrenia. PET also has the unique ability to allow the measurement of neurotransmitter release, which is well-characterised for dopamine and to a lesser extent endorphins.

One major advance that directly derived from PET studies was optimising the best and safest dose of drug treatments because the interactions of drugs with their receptor targets can be measured directly if there is a radiotracer that also binds to the receptor. This has been hugely useful in discovering if drugs were being dosed appropriately and so choosing the optimal dose to occupy the required number of brain receptor sites.

Once PET became available a number of brain-targeted medicines that had failed in clinical trials for unexplained reasons were found not to get into the brain! No target engagement means no chance of efficacy. Such drug-receptor occupation PET studies revolutionised the clinical pharmacology of drug treatments for schizophrenia. Before these human studies revealed the correct target dose of dopamine blocking drugs, many patients were being massively overdosed with consequent increases in adverse effects.

Both techniques allow us to perform serial measures on patients to monitor and discover disease progression and they have both been used to monitor brain function in non-affected relatives of people with disorders so allowing us to evaluate the genetic and familial contributions to them. PET but much more fMRI has shone a light into the silent and deep brain areas. They can measure activity in sub-cortical structures and many fMRI studies have shown the amygdala is activated by threatening images even without conscious awareness (subjective detection) of their content. This proves that this small brain region is a critical part of the rapid response fear reflex circuit.

Both PET and fMRI have demonstrated that the lower part of the basal ganglia (ventral striatum or also called the nucleus accumbens) is activated by motivated behaviour and the desire for some rewards, both of which probably are related to dopamine activity. The hidden secrets of the frontal lobes are being uncovered by fMRI studies of performance tasks that need thinking and attention with the lateral parts of the lobe being critical for high-level performance on these tasks. Also, the middle part of the frontal lobe, that part destroyed in Phineas Gage (*Chapter 3*), has now been shown to be active in thinking about oneself, planning behaviours and restraining others. It is also involved in responding to punishment and reward.

Perhaps the most impressive complementary discovery from independent PET and fMRI studies relates to the brain mechanisms of PTSD. Some sort of trauma has been experienced by almost everyone — we may have lost a parent or close friend, had a traffic accident or been assaulted. Initially the memory of the event is powerful usually with strong emotions as well. Over time this memory comes spontaneously into consciousness less often and then disappears unless something triggers its recall. But if the trauma has been significant enough it never goes entirely, at least not till our brain starts to degenerate as in dementia. This process of the brain slowly getting on top of traumatic memories is vital otherwise they would continue to bother us incessantly. But this is exactly what they do in patients with PTSD. Here they keep intruding in consciousness sometimes when provoked, e.g. by a sound or smell associated with the traumatic event, but often they emerge without any provocation and even in sleep this is very distracting to the person particularly if the emotional content of the trauma is strong as is typically the case with memories of being raped or blown-up in military conflict. So why are some people able to keep the memories at bay whilst others have them exploding into their minds on a regular basis?

The fMRI studies in groups of subjects that have experienced the same kinds and levels of traumas but in which some of them have developed PTSD and others haven't are revealing. They show that the difference lies in knowing to what extent the middle part of the frontal lobe (the medial prefrontal cortex or mPFC) is activated. This region suppresses traumatic memories and is more activated in the non-PTSD individuals than in those with PTSD.

So why do the PTSD patients fail to activate this region enough? PET studies reveal the answer, they have a deficit of GABA receptors in an adjacent region, just as in panic disorder where a failure of GABA inhibitory tone leads to a failure to stop panic attacks, and in epilepsy where a similar deficit leads to seizures, in PTSD a GABA failure leads to traumatic memory breakthroughs.

This is another example of how necessary the frontal lobe is to imposing top-down control of lower brain regions.

With the conflicts in the Middle-East, the Latin American drug wars and genocides in Africa, PTSD is becoming one the great challenges for modern psychiatry. As mentioned in *Chapter 2* serotonin-acting medications such as the SSRIs have some utility, but the majority of patients do not fully recover and many turn to alcohol and other drugs for solace that in medical terms tends to make things worse. Current psychotherapy treatment approaches emphasise the need to relive the trauma with a therapist in a secure and safe environment for a sufficient length of time that the accompanying emotional response eventually runs down (the emotion is extinguished). If this is done repeatedly the emotional side of the memory eventually fades so the person can talk about the factual elements of the trauma without having their thinking disrupted by flashbacks of emotion.

One new approach to this challenge is to combine drugs and psychotherapy so enabling the person to get control over the emotional elements more quickly. This can be done with pro-learning glutamate activating drugs such as D-cycloserine which has already proved useful in other fear disorders. The alternative strategy discussed already is to use one or two doses of the powerful anxiety and fear reducing drug MDMA alongside the psychotherapy. Several recent trials have shown this to work probably by releasing serotonin in areas of the brain such as the amygdala to dampen down fear so that the patient can recall the trauma without emotions overwhelming them.

Only dementia is able to fully eliminate the memory of a serious trauma, but sometimes, as dementia begins, PTSD memories can re-emerge after 40 or more years of lying dormant. Naturally, this often causes the person great distress. We were seeing a number of these cases of men who were traumatised in World War II and got over it. Then in their 80s and 90s, the memories they thought they had long-since overcome started re-emerging into consciousness. I think this occurs because as the brain ages it loses its capacity to continue suppressing the traumatic memories, so they break-out, just as they do at night during dreaming sleep when top-down cortical control of the emotional and memory centres is lessened.

Summary of Part I

- The evolution of the brain is one of the most remarkable aspects of life, arguably even more so than the evolution of DNA and of the cell as it has allowed humans to understand each of the other two major evolutionary developments and manipulate them for the benefit of our species.

- Brain development has taken several billions of years and involves that of protein pumps which can transmit ions into and out of the cell so creating the electrical gradients that drive neuronal activity.

- Other intracellular chemicals have become utilised as communication tools between neurons called neurotransmitters and some of these pumps have been modified to become neurotransmitter receptors whereas other receptors have developed from bacterial rhodopsin.

- The progressive growth of the brain has led to greater and greater power to regulate movement and other behaviours often at a reflex level. Also, the increase in its size has led to emergent properties such as consciousness. But remarkable as the brain is, it can, and indeed often does, go wrong.

In Part II of this book, we look at what happens when the brain does 'go wrong,' in particular, in relation to psychiatric and neurological disorders and consciousness.

PART II
ALTERED STATES OF MIND

CHAPTER 10

Sleep and Dreams

As we learned in *Chapter 1* the brain is a complex and sophisticated collection of billions of neurons that performs many different functions, some of which relate to self-awareness or consciousness. In this chapter we explore how consciousness is changed during sleep, and in medical and psychiatric disorders, with profound consequences for the person concerned and their family. Also, some people seek to alter their consciousness through changing their brain function with alcohol and other drugs and by changing their physiology, e.g. with carbon dioxide during (self-)asphyxiation for sexual pleasure. The reasons why we do this are complex and not well-researched but include novelty (one of the most powerful facets of the human brain is that it has a great hunger for new experiences), pleasure and fashion.

Even that small group of people who actively resist external means to alter consciousness all experience fundamental changes in consciousness every night when they sleep. Some people have profound experiences during dreams or nightmares or when they are falling into or coming out of sleep. Also doctors and other health professionals are often exposed to patients with profoundly altered states of consciousness. These range from those in the depths of depression who may in extreme cases feel that they are doing the Devil's work or have the Devil inside them, to patients with mania who believe they are God (or some other deity). I have seen people with schizophrenia, dementias or brain tumours develop completely different personalities to the horror of their families though with no insight themselves of how they have changed.

Most health professionals will have tried to help people with an infection who have developed delirium and are behaving well out of character. Sometimes this can include attacking the staff trying to help them. But when the infection is treated, and they recover, they have no recollection of that behaviour. I explained in the *Introduction* how when working as an emergency GP I was fought off by a diabetic man with extreme life-threateningly low blood sugar levels (hypoglycaemia). He had no insight that without my intervention he would likely die. With his wife's help I held him down and managed to give him an intravenous injection of glucose. We then both watched in relief and wonder as he returned to normal consciousness in seconds, but with no recollection of his violent opposition just a minute before. Similarly, I have seen patients with epilepsy fit in front of me with no recollection of their behaviour when they came round. One man with temporal lobe epilepsy (partial complex seizures) wandered around the room to a different spot while rubbing his nose and then when he recovered asked us why we had moved.

How can brain science help us make sense of these profound and often frightening alterations in consciousness? And what do they tell us about how the mind and brain work? I think more than we often suppose, because there are so many different sorts of these experiences ranging from sleep to delirium.

Everyone sleeps — Almost everyone

We all sleep, though often less than we would like; sleep is an essential part of the daily (circadian) cycle of life. All animals sleep to some extent, often in short episodes, although humans have developed a strong consolidation of sleep, so that we largely do it once only and during the night or dark period of each 24 hours. We are therefore diurnal animals and this sleep pattern distinguishes us from nocturnal animals such as cats and mice that tend to sleep in the day and be active at night.

We know sleep is vital for life because if we don't have enough of it we get ill. Experience with torture and interrogation methods including sleep deprivation have shown that the latter kills people faster than either water or food deprivation; in the stressful environment of a prison with interrogation, sleep deprivation of more than a few nights can be lethal. But also sleep deprivation can be useful. Staying awake overnight can help to lift mood in a depressed person although the antidepressant benefit is lost once they fall asleep again.

This further confirms our understanding that depression is a biological process that either exerts itself on top of normal mood function or emerges when normal mood cannot be sustained. Religious experiences also can emerge from sleep deprivation. Long periods of overnight prayer, often with a degree of pain from kneeling, were used by monks and knights pre-the Crusades as a way of achieving insights into faith. Sleep deprivation commonly leads to visions (visual hallucinations) and sometimes to hearing things (auditory hallucinations). These may develop a meaning to the person particularly if they are being actively sought-after. As with other forms of deprivation discussed below sleep deprivation is thought to produce physiological and metabolic alterations in the brain that allow these hallucinations to develop.

Sleep is not a passive process, the brain doesn't just switch-off or shut down, in fact it may at times, particularly during rapid eye movement (REM) (dreaming) sleep, be more active and use more energy than it does when the dreamer is awake. As any insomniac will tell you sleep can be a hard state to achieve. In my sleep clinic I used to compare overcoming insomnia with playing golf—both sleep and good golf are harder to achieve the more you try! Sleep occurs because of a subconscious active process that switches-off arousal systems in the brain. Many insomniacs find it doesn't happen as quickly as they would like because they are chronically over-aroused. In this way they are the opposite of patients with narcolepsy, in whom, as we saw in *Chapter 7*, this turning-off of the arousal systems occurs too easily.

The switching-off of the brain that is required for sleep occurs as a result of two separate brain processes coming together, usually at the start of the night. One is the basic rhythm of the brain over its 24 hour (circadian) cycle that is in part-controlled by the hormone melatonin. We rarely feel this rhythm until we change our time zones and then get the experience of jet lag. This rhythm makes it hard to go to sleep when we go east and hard to wake-up when we go west. The other sleep driver is the 'pressure' to sleep that increases the longer we are awake. This process is driven by metabolic products of the brain such as adenosine that are explained below. When both processes are in synchrony sleep comes relatively easily but if they are out of phase, e.g. with jet lag or shift work then it is much harder to get to sleep.

Most cases of insomnia are due to excessive arousal probably produced by excess release of neurotransmitters such as noradrenaline; this is called physiological insomnia and can be treated with hypnotics (sleeping pills) such as benzodiazepines or by relaxation training. Some people suffer from a weakness of the circadian drive, and these are harder to help though melatonin administration may help a little if given at the correct part of the evening.

The purpose of sleep is still something of a mystery to science (see below). But one thing is certain — we all know that if we are deprived of a night's sleep, or have even just have a couple of hours less than usual, then we feel tired and irritable and underperform the next day. Persistent total sleep deprivation will eventually lead to death. We see this with rare brain syndromes that result in an inability to sleep and lead to premature death. One is fatal familial insomnia where a genetic mutation leads to progressive damage to the sleep-promoting areas of the brain so that the ability to sleep is progressively reduced and eventually is completely lost, with death occurring soon after despite the best efforts of doctors.

I had one patient with this disorder, a middle-aged man whose insomnia continued to break through every dose of sleep-promoting medicines I prescribed. Over a few months, despite heroic doses, his lack of sleep killed him. Some patients with extreme mania also stay awake for days and then die as a result. In most of these cases of severe insomnia the deaths are usually the result of a stress-induced cardiac event.

These syndromes of severe insomnia tell us that sleep is vital to life and also that it is an active process that can be damaged (as in familial insomnia) or overridden (as in mania). During sleep we rest our muscles, and this is probably restorative to them as they are particularly relaxed during dreaming sleep when the neuronal outputs from the brain to the muscles are switched-off. Also, in the first few hours of sleep the hypothalamus secretes growth hormone that helps the body grow and restore itself. The levels of some other hormones, e.g. cortisol, fall during sleep and then rise again as we wake-up.

Recently work in mice has suggested that during sleep there is an increase in the flow of fluid around the brain that may serve to 'flush out' unwanted products of brain activity so allowing restoration of function the next day. Certainly, the sleepiness that occurs as the day wears on is induced in part by the build-up of breakdown products from brain metabolism, particularly adenosine. This small molecule acts on specialised adenosine receptors in the brain to switch-off some of the awake-maintaining neurotransmitters such as histamine, so we begin to feel sleepy.

The ability of coffee to keep us awake is because the active ingredient of this drink—caffeine—is a blocker of the adenosine receptor, so stops the sedative action of adenosine. The use of caffeine in many 'energy' drinks is based on this fact, that it helps offset sleep so users can stay awake for longer. Because caffeine is alerting it is now commonplace for young people to use caffeine-containing soft drinks to offset the sedative effects of alcohol, so allowing them to drink more or for longer. Other stimulants do the same and the drink-fuelled rowdy exploits of the Oxford Bullingdon Club were allegedly conducted on the back of cocaine intake that kept members awake and probably also contributed to their sometimes ostensibly violent behaviour.

Sleep is a mixture of different states of consciousness but at no point does the brain become unconscious in the sense that is seen during coma or anaesthesia. We know this because mental events such as dreams happen during sleep, and ongoing computational activity is revealed by experiences such as the brain keeping track of time. It never ceases to amaze me how well the brain computes time during sleep to (usually) wake me up just before the alarm clock goes off!

Sometimes sleep seems to open-up new avenues of problem solving—hence the expression 'sleep on it.' A very famous example is that of the well-known German organic chemist August Kekulé (1829–1896) who was struggling with the structure of a new molecule he had identified that resembled hexene but had two fewer hydrogen atoms. One night when he dropped-off in front of his fireplace he awoke suddenly with the realisation that instead of being a straight chain like hexene the molecule was circular in structure, i.e. the two ends of the chain were joined; the molecule was cyclo-hexene which we now know as the 'benzene ring.' This sleep-related insight laid the foundation of all modern organic chemistry.

Stages of sleep

The early stages of sleep (Stages 1 and 2) occur as one drops-off. Awareness of the environment begins to decrease though we can still hear conversations particularly if they relate to us. In these stages people sometimes experience a sense of falling as their muscles relax. In some cases, this can be associated with other odd perceptions such as visual hallucinations (called hypnogogic hallucinations) that can be distressing and wake-up the incipient sleeper. Sometimes fear of these 'attacks' leads to anxiety about falling sleeping which in turn results in insomnia.

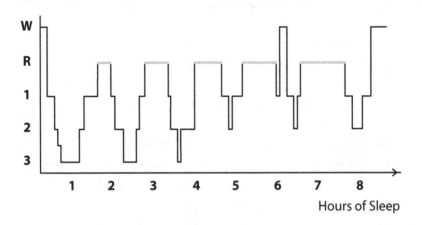

Figure 10: The stages of sleep across the
night — Normal hypnogram (R = REM sleep)

After some minutes in these lighter stages the person descends into the deeper stages of sleep (Stages 3 and 4) and loses contact with the outside world. These deep stages are maximal in the early part of the night and during them the brain is in a very synchronised state with the EEG showing slow and deep activity, which give these stages the alternative name slow wave sleep (SWS). This is the sleep stage when growth hormone is released and is thought to be the most necessary part of sleep. We believe this for several reasons. One is that SWS comes early in the night so is the stage least likely to be lost by insomnia. The other reason is that when people are totally sleep deprived then in their catch-up sleep, the next night, they have increased amounts of this deep sleep.

Following the first SWS period that can last up to 60 minutes the person then moves into a short period of the lighter stages of sleep from which the first episode of dreaming sleep (rapid eye movement or REM sleep) happens.

REM sleep used to be called paradoxical sleep because the EEG recordings show a waking-type of pattern—yet people were asleep! However, in REM sleep muscle activity is very low as the brain suppresses spinal cord activity. This suppression is believed to assist in restoring muscle function, but it also serves a critical role in limiting the ability of us to act on our dreams. We shall learn later that when this muscle suppression breaks down strange and unpleasant episodes of behaviour can occur called REM behaviour disorder.

Night terrors and sleepwalking

Most sleep-related behaviours occur out of deep (SWS) sleep, most commonly night terrors and sleepwalking. These are common in children (about 25% have some sort of episode) but can persist into adulthood in about one per cent of the population. They run in families and I have treated three generations of one family with this disorder. Further evidence of a genetic link is given by the high incidence of them in people of Welsh descent in towns in Patagonia, presumably due to a founder effect from an affected individual settling there and siring many children and grandchildren who all had the same (as yet unidentified) genetic mutation.

The cause of these deep sleep related phenomena (also called confusional arousals) isn't fully understood. They are thought to be due to some waking-up of subcortical brain structures, maybe from anxiety, while the cortex is still asleep. The person is therefore unconscious in the sense that they have no awareness and hence no memory of what is arousing them, but their more primitive parts of the brain, e.g. the amygdala, act on these experiences usually with fear reflexes.

With night terrors sufferers often sit-up in bed and scream, but unless woken-up have no recollection of what was frightening them. If they are woken, they usually describe a sense of dread or terror of something large, threatening and frightening being in the room. These attacks are very distressing to partners and others sharing accommodation with the person as they usually occur when they are also asleep; the scream wakes them up thinking the person screaming is being attacked. This causes further anxiety to their partner or others in the house and significant embarrassment in the sufferer, and it is often this that leads them to seek help.

On rare occasions some sufferers from night terrors have more formed hallucinations. One patient of mine who when sleeping in a tent in a forest in Europe with a friend thought he was being attacked by a bear, feeling the animals claws around his throat. To escape the clutches of the bear he bit what his hallucinating brain told him was the bear's paw but was in fact his friend's hand. He was then woken by the scream of his tent-mate whose hand he had deeply injured. The friend had been woken-up by the night terror scream and had tried to wake his frightened but still-sleeping friend only to be badly bitten for his efforts!

Night terrors come from deep sleep which is usually thought of as being relatively low in conscious activity, but clearly there are cognitive processes going on. They are not necessarily always fearful or threatening, but when they are fear-related they can result in screaming with terror and escape attempts. These phenomena come from activity in the amygdala that coordinates fear responses in the awake state by orchestrating the necessary range of responses from screams to warn others, increases in heart rate and breathing, and escape responses.

Sleepwalking is a related phenomenon but usually without a scream of terror. The person starts to move and walk around the bedroom often with a worried or quizzical look on their face. Sometimes they engage in work-related behaviour as with a patient of mine who would lay out all his tools for the next day's work on the floor then return to bed and wake the next morning with no recollection of why the tools were on the floor. More commonly the sleepwalker tries to get out of the room, opening doors and windows. Sometimes they succeed in leaving the bedroom and wander off into other parts of the house or beyond. This can lead them to harm, and it's been estimated maybe ten or so deaths per year in the UK result from sleepwalkers falling off stairs and balconies. This is more likely when in a strange bedroom and when drunk, which explains why these episodes are common in Mediterranean holiday resorts popular with young people.

In one well-reported case of sleepwalking the person woke-up to find himself halfway down a cliff. Not only did he have no recollection of how he got there but also was unable to climb back, needing to be rescued by the emergency services. In my clinical practice I would commonly advise my patients to take extra door and window locks on vacation—and to hide the key so they can't open these during a sleepwalking episode.

These phenomena and those of nightmares (discussed in the next section) tell us that a degree of organized mental activity that would be considered conscious if the patient was awake can occur with no memory or awareness if the person is in deep sleep. The best explanation is that the key wake centres of the cortex are still switched off, so the patient is asleep whilst other brain regions, e.g. the brain stem and hippocampus are functioning normally. Hence the person can walk and even talk a bit but isn't aware of what they are doing, and so can't lay down any memory of it. However, the repetitive processes that sleepwalkers engage in often reflect their normal concerns when awake. A good example is those cases of people who are on restricted diets who seek out food by making their way to the kitchen or fridge and stuffing themselves during the night before returning to bed. The only evidence of their nocturnal excursions the half-emptied fridge and the mess they leave behind in the kitchen.

The reason why some parts of the brain are awake but others not is beginning to be understood. Brain arousal and wakefulness is driven by a small set of neurons in the brain stem that project to most of the rest of the brain and activate it. At a certain level of activation, the cortex wakes-up and we realise we are awake. However, if the cortex doesn't wake-up then the rest of the brain can do its thing without us being aware of it. In children the arousal drive that leads to sleepwalking is usually a full bladder. Often the child slips back into quiet sleep once they have peed.

In adults, a full bladder may provoke attacks but more often is seems to be that ongoing cognitive processes, usually ones of worry, can lead to sleepwalking. We know this because sometimes people wake-up fully during an episode and can describe their feelings. Also sleepwalking is more common when people are psychologically stressed or aroused by other factors, e.g. taking caffeine or eating chocolate or cheese before going to bed. Some of my patients would eliminate all stimulants from their diet after lunchtime to protect against this. Also, they would avoid watching scary movies in the evenings as the frightening images from these seemed to resonate in their brains despite their being asleep and lead to more night terrors or sleepwalking.

Drugs can aggravate or even allow sleepwalking to occur. The most common culprit is alcohol which increases deep sleep early in the night, and so provides more time in SWS for these behaviours to occur. Many people who sleepwalk avoid alcohol for this reason. Sometimes extremely violent behaviour can occur during sleepwalking episodes, and these may be magnified by alcohol's aggression-promoting actions.

In some cases, sleepwalking is used as a defence in murder cases, though when alcohol has been involved it may be hard to prove. With the exception of cases where the accused has a long-proven history of sleepwalking and related behaviours, or where the defendant has PTSD from military exposure and so may be reacting to earlier near-death experiences, trial juries tend to err in favour of convicting the accused.

I was once involved as an expert witness in one case of death from multiple stabbings of a very drunk person by an equally highly intoxicated alcoholic housemate during the early hours of one morning. At court he claimed that as he had no memory of the attack he must have been sleepwalking. But with no prior proven episodes, and a rather systematic knife assault having been carried out, the jury's decision was one of manslaughter. My analysis was that it was more likely that the amnesia was due to extreme alcohol intoxication than sleepwalking.

Another drug linked to sleepwalking is zolpidem. This is a newer hypnotic (sleeping-pill) that specifically targets the α_1 subtype of GABA-A receptors in the cortex, through which it switches-off cortical activity. This promotes sleep but because zolpidem doesn't suppress the sub-cortical systems as much as typical benzodiazepine sleeping pills such as temazepam, these systems may be more easily aroused and lead to sleepwalking whilst the zolpidem still keeps the cortex asleep.

Despite their being relatively common particularly in children there is little research into the treatment of night terrors and sleepwalking with many adult sufferers finding their GPs are dismissive or even amused by their tales. Reducing anxiety at night using the approaches mentioned already, e.g. no caffeine, avoiding large late meals and scary films, can help in milder cases. For more severe ones, particularly those where people have put themselves at risk, then anxiolytic drugs such as a broad-acting benzodiazepine (e.g. clonazepam) or a serotonin promoting drug such as an SSRI can be very effective and may stop a sequence of bad nights. They can be very helpful for patients who are at high risk of attacks when sleeping away from home, e.g. can be taken prophylactically for the first week at a camp or when starting at university.

Dreams and nightmares

EEG recordings of sleep show almost everyone dreams but many people have little or no memory of their dreams' contents so believe they don't dream. Nightmares are dreams with unpleasant or frightening images and as the content tends to wake up the dreamer they are usually better remembered than more pleasant dreams. But if people who deny dreaming are woken during REM sleep, they will remember dreaming at least for a short while. In some cultures dreams are seen as highly valuable experiences and so methods to induce and remember them are developed and encouraged. A similar approach is also used by some psychotherapists belonging to Freudian and Jungian schools as they believe that the content of dreams can help identify issues the patient is struggling with. Proving the value of this approach to therapy is not easy but every psychiatrist knows that the content of dreams changes dramatically during episodes of mental illness, particularly in depression when frightening and anxious themes dominate.

The prominence of dreaming in depression probably reflects the fact that the amount of time spent in REM sleep increases in this mood state, possibly due to a deficit of serotonin, one of the neurotransmitters that normally limit dreaming. Antidepressants that increase serotonin like the SSRIs have the opposite effect and markedly suppress REM sleep. In manic states dreams may be of empowerment and success but may be of depressive content too, supporting the analysts' view that the elevated mood of mania can be a defence against prior or incipient depression.

There is other evidence that dreams do reflect awake mental states particularly those the person is heavily engaged in. Many of us will have dreamed about exams or other stressful forthcoming events. I still vividly recall dreaming I had failed all my A-levels a month before the exam; luckily this premonition was wrong! When people are intensively engaged for a period in activities they often dream about them, e.g. stamp collecting, sewing or even for academics writing grant applications!

We can use the fact that the contents of waking consciousness are able to influence dreams to assist people with recurrent nightmares. The approach is to get them to recount the nightmare. Usually these wake them when something terrible is about to happen, e.g. they are being chased and fall off a cliff. We then get them to choose and write down a happy ending, e.g. they jump off the cliff but land on a boat that the pursing creatures can't access, and the boat then sails away to a wonderful and peaceful tropical island. They then rehearse this ending and remarkably it often gets incorporated into the dream sequence. At least that's what we think happens as the nightmare no longer wakens them so we can't be sure it still happens with the different ending.

The most damaging nightmares are those that occur as a result of trauma as in PTSD where frightening memories of the trauma can occur every night or even several times a night. Naturally, this is horribly distressing to the traumatised person as it continues to force the memory of the trauma into their consciousness. Moreover, at night they are often alone with no-one to support them. And even if with a partner the nightmare awakenings can still be very distressing and put a huge strain on this relationship (well-illustrated in the 2013 film of a soldier traumatised in a Japanese prisoner of War Camp, 'The Railway Man').

In addition, the sleep disruption caused by the repeated awakenings from nightmares, and the mental arousal they produce making going back to sleep difficult, leads to great psychological distress, physical stress, and often depression. As I have already noted elsewhere, for military personnel trained to respond to enemy assault, these nightmares may involve reliving being under attack and so they can lash out and attack their bed partners thinking they are the enemy, sometimes with painful or even lethal consequences.

'To sleep ... perchance to dream'

This line from Hamlet's soliloquy 'To be or not to be ...' in the play of the same name sums up a key question—what is the purpose of dreams? In the 400 years since William Shakespeare wrote it this remains a fundamental question but one into which we have little insight still.

We know that REM sleep is probably useful though cannot be entirely sure of this as there are patients on strong antidepressants, particularly the MOAIs like phenelzine, who seem to live quite comfortably despite having little or no REM for many years, since these medicines suppress REM very powerfully. We also know that depriving people of REM sleep leads to some catch up the next night though not as much as occurs when SWS is deprived (above).

On the other hand, the strong link between dream content and ongoing daytime activities and mental issues clearly suggests that some processing of daytime learning is taking place. A lot of rodent work, with some human experiments suggesting the same, has found that certain aspects of memory are enhanced by REM sleep. So, people will perform better on tasks learned just before sleep if they have good quality REM rather than if it is disrupted.

The failure of PTSD nightmares to resolve matters is one of the major challenges to the idea that REM sleep is about sorting out problems, though it may be that the images of PTSD are just too extreme and profound to be dealt with at a subcortical level of processing. Another challenge to this idea is the syndrome of REM behaviour disorder, a condition that is becoming more common as overnight sleep EEG studies show it to be quite different from sleepwalking though the outward appearance is very similar. In essence REM behaviour disorder is a syndrome of acting out dreams, or more usually nightmares.

During most people's REM sleep there is muscle paralysis, possibly to allow muscle energy restoration but also to stop people acting on their dream content. Imagine if every time we had a dream of being chased we started running, sleep would be a very unsatisfying and even dangerous experience. REM sleep is characterised by extreme muscle relaxation with only the eye muscles able to break free from this paralysis, hence the term rapid eye movement (REM) sleep, as the eyes move to some extent. Studies with those rare people who have lucid dreaming, i.e. are able to dream and relate the content in a continuous fashion, have found the eye movements during REM are mostly tracking movements of the eyes following the images moving in the dream. However, in some people, most commonly middle-aged men, the muscle paralysis of REM sleep begins to break down and they start to act out their dreams. As with night terrors this is mostly seen when the dreams are frightening and threatening, and the patient reacts with anger and violence. Patients of mine have smashed bedside lights and tables believing them to be people attacking them, and even on occasions punched through walls in self-defence. This is naturally a worry to their bed partners who may themselves be attacked and so often move into a separate room.

Recently it has become apparent that REM behaviour disorder is due to the failure of the dopamine system in the brain. It is therefore a forerunner of Parkinson's disease that emerges five or more years later as more of the dopamine neurons in the brain die. Why a loss of dopamine leads to violent nightmares and loss of muscle paralysis in REM is not known but treatments that increase dopamine like L-DOPA can help reduce the number and severity of attacks of this sleep disorder. Making more doctors aware of it is now important as if diagnosed early it may offer a chance to intervene and so slow the progression of Parkinson's disease.

At the other end of the REM muscle paralysis spectrum are those people who have too much paralysis usually manifest by their waking-up before the paralysis has been switched-off. They experience a phenomenon called sleep paralysis that is very distressing as for a short while they realise they are paralysed and have no way of knowing if they will ever move again! Of course, they do, usually within a few seconds of waking, but the fear of another paralysis the next night can be very distressing and lead to insomnia. It is not uncommon for people with this disorder to resort to the use of alcohol and other sedative drugs to overcome their fear of sleep with a likely waking from sleep with paralysis.

Sleep paralysis is associated with visual hallucinations as well and both are due to the REM system staying active for a few moments during wakefulness; normally waking switches it off. These experiences are not uncommon, probably 30 per cent or more of the population have had them at least once in their life. They are more likely when sleep patterns are disturbed, e.g. with jet lag or shift work (which explains their colloquial name of 'night-nurse paralysis' as nurses sleeping in the day after a night shift would commonly report them). The paralysis can be aborted by a simple touch to the hand or foot by a bed partner if it doesn't stop spontaneously. This probably is due to sensory touch information activating the muscle arousal systems that are still switched-off.

In some rare cases I have treated patients who have many of these episodes each night. They usually sleep alone so have no-one to help them out of the paralysis. They may lay paralysed for minutes, though this feels like hours, and often report extreme muscle exhaustion the next day, probably as a consequence of the massive mental efforts they make in trying to move their frozen muscles. One patient of mine who had two-to-four attacks each night said each one was like pulling himself up to the ceiling on the curtains using just his arms.

Dreams and consciousness

Dreams and other sleep-related experiences raise intriguing questions for our understanding of consciousness. In most cases they are a form of consciousness without a memory of the content being laid down. This is probably because the same processes that are required for cortex arousal and waking are also critical in laying down memories. However, if there is arousal from dreams, as occurs usually at the end of the night's sleep or with nightmares, then memories of the dream content can be encoded.

Some people are very good at remembering their dreams and a few with lucid dreaming have the ability to recount dreams as they go along. This tells us that the content of dreams is amenable to consciousness awareness in some cases, and lucid dreamers may even be able to direct their content to some extent.

The most obviously similar altered consciousness state to dreaming is that seen with the psychedelic state. EEG and brain imaging studies have shown that the temporal lobes and hippocampus are active in this state, and psychedelics can induce dreaming if injected intravenously during other stages of sleep. In both states, reality is changed with strange and sometimes wonderful images experienced. But also in both states fear and terror can occur if the person is anxious or frightened or has another psychiatric disorder. The main difference is that normally the cortex is awake during the psychedelic experience and asleep during dreaming.

The fact that violent and fearful images in nightmares, night terrors and REM behaviour disorder, three very different stages of sleep, occur and are so common raises interesting questions for the human psyche about whether because the role of violence is so common it would emerge in all us if we had these disorders. Or is it just that the acting out of responses to violent threats makes it more likely that people wake-up and so report the violent images? To separate these two options, we would need to wake people with these disorders multiple times at different stages of sleep and explore their dream content. This would be a challenging set of studies and so they have not yet been conducted.

CHAPTER 11

In Extremis — Near Death Experiences and Vegetative States

I n the previous chapter we discussed the neurotransmitters and brain regions involved in maintaining arousal and wakefulness. Glutamate and other neurotransmitters such as noradrenaline, histamine and orexin keep you awake, GABA puts you to sleep (as also do drugs that block the wake-promoting neurotransmitters such as antihistamines). We also considered the strange, altered state of locked-in syndrome where movement isn't possible, but consciousness can be probed using imaging techniques.

There are other medical disorders that can lead to profound alterations of consciousness and so can help us gain a better understanding of brain mechanisms. One of these is the near-death experience that is seen when people come close to death or are even believed to have died as a result, e.g. of a heart attack. When they are brought back to life or recover unaided, they commonly describe experiences of floating out of their body into the air and so being able to look down on their body below. Another frequent report is of seeing a very bright white light in the centre of their vision like a massive star that can seem to draw them towards it.

In some cases, this can be like a palace or temple in a distant city or on a hill. The floating out-of-body experience is remarkably common and is usually interpreted by the patient as their 'soul' leaving their body for a short while. There have been attempts to test this scientifically by putting special signs on the top of cupboards in intensive care units so that only something/someone floating above them would be able to see it. The knowledge of these signs was then tested when the patients had recovered and left the ward but no evidence of any memory of these was obtained. This is not surprising as the scientific evidence for a soul is lacking. What seems much more likely is that the out-of-body experience is something generated in the brain as it approaches death due to lack of oxygen or glucose.

It seems possible that the biblical claim that 'In the beginning was the light' might come from this observation that all that's left at the end of life is the light. When all other capacities in the brain fail, complex images in the real and imagined world cannot be constructed and so all that is left is for the visual system to see unformed light. Some people in the psychedelic state also have this sense of a strong vital light in the distance like a celestial city or a great star. These visions may reflect a breakdown of standard visual processing pathways so that only light, not form or colour or movement, is processed. Then the memory circuits of the brain take over and images that may be real, imagined or taken from literature, art, cinema or religion (as per the example below), may emerge into consciousness and then be remembered.

An intriguing example of this state is given by the US neurosurgeon Eben Alexander in his book *Proof of Heaven: A Neurosurgeon's Journey into the Afterlife* (see *Selected Bibliography*). He was a successful surgeon with a stable family life until he contracted a virulent form of bacterial meningitis with a high likelihood of dying. Luckily, he was in a quality medical centre and the diagnosis was made before it was too late and treatment was initiated. Nevertheless, for several weeks he was in coma and near to death. Gradually he recovered and then with great relief and thankful to the God he met in his near-death state he told the world of his trip to Heaven in his book.

In essence, for several weeks when not conscious of the outside world due to the meningitis, Alexander travelled through some form of space. Initially this was a bleak dark place rather mud-like and filled with worms but as the days passed the environment got lighter and, at some point, he felt as if he had entered Heaven. The book was a best-seller on the *New York Times* list, and he became a celebrity.

His experience is not unique and similar out-of-body experiences have been reported by many people with life threatening illnesses, and also others who have put themselves through major alterations in health, e.g. through fasting or sleep deprivation. This concept of altering the mind to find God through metabolic challenges is millennia old. The most famous case of all was of course that of Jesus Christ who used what was probably a common approach by ascetics at that time of starvation to induce mystical experiences.

It is extremely unlikely that Jesus actually starved for 40 days and 40 nights since this is not compatible with life. But even a couple of weeks starvation will lead to significant changes in blood chemistry and glucose deprivation that would profoundly alter brain function. With nothing to eat he would have first used up the body's stores of carbohydrate which are mostly in the form of glycogen in the liver to provide glucose for the brain and muscle. Over the first week this would have been depleted then his body would have started to break down fat stores for energy.

Breaking down fat with little/no carbohydrate results in the production of high levels of metabolic products called ketone bodies. These change the acid-base balance of the brain, and this alters brain function. Sometimes we use this high fat (so-called ketogenic) diet in children with intractable epilepsy that doesn't respond to anti-convulsant medicines. We don't exactly know how this works but in some of my first experiments I showed that in rats this diet has a profound impact on GABA function in the brain which is probably how it stops seizures. However, when coupled with low blood glucose the ketone bodies would begin to impair cognitive function.

Eventually Jesus' fat stores would be entirely used up, so his muscles would begin to break down the protein in their fibres to keep the heart and brain energy supplies up. The protein breakdown would result in raised levels of substances such as ammonia that can profoundly alter brain function. After a couple of weeks, a form of delirium would emerge with visual and other hallucinations and sleep disruption almost inevitable. In the prepared mind of Jesus, who was deliberately starving himself to facilitate communication with God, the destabilisation of the regular brain state would facilitate the emergence of new experiences and beliefs. These would break down the brain's typical resistance to change the way it perceives things. This less rigid state of brain function would facilitate his efforts, intentions and prior beliefs to become more certain of his relationship with his God. At some point revelation would have occurred when Jesus suddenly realised he was God's son, i.e. Jesus Christ, with a vital mission to fulfil on Earth.

A similar 'toxic' experience seems to have underpinned the development of the Baha'i faith. This is the most recent of the Judaeo-Christian religions founded in the 19th century by Baha'u'llah. The name Baha'i means 'of glory' and this religion is generally seen as a development of Shia Islam though with inputs from many other world religions. The prophet Baha'u'llah was persecuted by the State and kept imprisoned for many years in chains with sleep deprivation and starvation. Whilst in this period of stress and deprivation he experienced visions:

> 'During the days I lay in the prison of Tihran, though the galling weight of the chains and the stench-filled air allowed Me but little sleep, still in those infrequent moments of slumber I felt as if something flowed from the crown of My head over My breast, even as a mighty torrent that precipitateth itself upon the earth from the summit of a lofty mountain. Every limb of My body would, as a result, be set afire. At such moments My tongue recited what no man could bear to hear.'

In delirium, weird images appear and interestingly, despite the metabolic poisoning of the brain, sometimes they are remembered, probably when they are of sufficient meaning or strangeness.

Once when I was a junior doctor, I became delirious with sunstroke and I suddenly developed a paranoid delusion. I became certain that I'd made a major mistake in my practice and that my career would be over because people already knew. The next morning when I had recovered the fear had dissipated but my factual memory of the event and the content of the paranoia persists to this day. Again, this is reminiscent of the psychedelic state and there is some evidence that psychedelic-like substances may be produced in some infections that cause delirium. Also, the stress of infections can produce chemical messengers called cytokines that directly affect brain function and alter serotonin metabolism and so may predispose this altered state of consciousness.

CHAPTER 12

Affliction of the Gods? — Epilepsy

After sleep and drug use, epilepsy is probably the most well-known form of altered consciousness. Most people have seen someone have a *grand mal* fit in which they lose consciousness and experience a series of muscle spasms with facial grimacing and sometimes loss of bladder control. In ancient times such seizures were seen as an indication of visitation from the gods and those people with epilepsy were often thought to have special powers and were accorded special status.

The fit was seen as a direct interaction with the gods. Caesar Augustus (Julius Caesar) who became an Emperor of Rome and then a 'God' was one such person who benefited from having the divine affliction of epilepsy. He also benefited from having a shock of red hair (that he was named after) as this was also seen as giving special powers. Many other less dramatic forms of epilepsy exist ranging from episodes of absence seizures to the aforementioned *grand mal* seizures. Absence seizures (also called *petit mal* fits) in children may be so transient that they go unnoticed by parents or teachers for years, or are misinterpreted as deliberate inattention or laziness.

Complex partial seizures are the most common form of epilepsy and also go by the name 'temporal lobe epilepsy.' They occur because inside the temporal lobe the hippocampus has become damaged, usually as a result of a long-lasting seizure that deprives this part of the brain of oxygen, that then results in neuronal damage. This damage becomes a scar that is deficient in the inhibitory neurotransmitter GABA and so more seizures occur.

In most cases the initial damage is caused by a febrile seizure in childhood. These are quite common seizures that happen when a child has a high fever and there is a genetic predisposition to these. If they last for over 30 minutes then the hippocampus can be damaged. In many cases subsequent seizures do not emerge until adolescence though in more severely affected children the epilepsy can start soon after the first seizure.

Temporal lobe epilepsy is associated with many brain phenomena other than seizures which make it a veritable goldmine for students of consciousness and perception. Often the seizures start with an altered sense of smell or taste or a feeling of warmth in the abdomen or chest or of anxiety. These are called 'auras' as they warn that a seizure is about to happen unless something is done to abort it (e.g. giving an anti-epilepsy drug). These auras reflect activation of brain regions in the temporal lobe near to the epilepsy focus. Feelings of anxiety are thought to be due to amygdala activity, warmth from the insula, smell and taste from the olfactory lobes. These activities may be part of the seizure or may be a local side-effect neuronal response to the incipient seizure in an attempt to stop it.

Many temporal lobe epilepsy attacks are predominantly behavioural in nature so are often mistaken for other forms of odd behaviour such as drunkenness, insolence, drug intoxication and forms of mental-illness, especially psychosis. This is particularly likely for seizures that last a long time. In some cases, temporal lobe seizures may go on for hours without treatment because doctors do not realise that the behaviour may be a form of seizure.

A good example from my clinical experience is having seen the police called to deal with a difficult man in casualty who wouldn't listen to the nursing staff and was spitting repeatedly and turning his head away from them. Before the police got involved temporal lobe epilepsy was diagnosed and the administration of an IV dose of the anti-epilepsy drug diazepam rapidly brought him out of his seizure and back to normal. Without this diagnosis having been made he could have been taken into custody and suffered irretrievable brain damage from the prolonged untreated seizure.

It is all too common for people with odd behaviour from conditions such as epilepsy and schizophrenia to get arrested and taken into police custody where they may come to more harm. The most ridiculous and disappointing case I heard of recently was as a man with dementia who would not stop wandering around the hospital being arrested for disturbing the peace!

Other more complex behavioural actions and sensory experiences may appear with temporal lobe epilepsy. One of the most intriguing is fugues where the patient wanders off for hours or even days. In these periods of altered consciousness new ideas and experiences may emerge and be acted upon. It has been suggested by at least one eminent neurologist that the wanderings of the prophet Mohammed that led to his interactions with God might have been due to his having this form of epilepsy. Some of the descriptions of how he was during these inspirational episodes are strongly reminiscent of temporal lobe epilepsy. Quotes such as:

'Those who saw the Prophet in this state relate that his condition would change. Sometimes he would stay motionless as if some terribly heavy load was pressed on him and, even in the coldest day, drops of sweat would fall from his forehead, at other times he would move his lips.'

And also:

'At the moment of inspiration, anxiety pressed upon the Prophet, and his countenance was troubled.'

'He fell to the ground like one intoxicated or overcome by sleep. Inspiration descended unexpectedly, and without any previous warning.'

Certainly, in my clinical practice I have seen individuals with temporal lobe damage develop extreme alterations in beliefs such that they disown their families and become very different in personality and attitude. This is different to the facile personality changes seen in frontal lobe lesions (as in the tale of Phineas Gage: *Chapter 3*) as the behaviour is more formulated and not impulsive but equally resistant to reasoning.

CHAPTER 13

Darkness Visible? Depression

D epression and anxiety are the most common brain disorders, affecting up to 40 per cent of Western populations over a lifetime. Most families know someone who had — or is currently suffering from — these disorders. The burden to society of the two together is the costliest of all medical disorders, even more than cancer and heart disease. They can take many different forms, with varying degrees of severity. Their impact can range from a change in mental state that is disturbing but still permits the person to live a nearly normal life, to deep depressions that can lead the sufferer to become immobile and incapable of even eating or drinking or severe anxiety that makes them housebound through agoraphobia (a fear of going out).

Very often depression and anxiety go together, usually with anxiety preceding the depression. One view is that depression emerges from chronic anxiety as a form of mental exhaustion. Anxiety is a defensive reaction that helps protect the person from threat, either physical or psychological. It involves increased levels of arousal and alertness, often with sleep disruption (insomnia: *Chapter 10*) and increased motor activity such as pacing and handwringing or hair twisting.

Eventually, after a period of intense anxiety that may last for months or years the brain's arousal systems begin to deplete and then depression with its characteristic lack of drive and energy takes over. Thought content in anxiety is about future threats and how to deal with them, whereas in depression the thought content becomes about current and past failures. However, if the thought processes are not discovered by the medical profession and only the peripheral somatic symptoms such as pain and fatigue are considered then the underlying psychiatric problem can be missed with costly unnecessary medical interventions and harmful results.

In my 40 years of psychiatric practice, I have seen very many people with depression so choosing patients stories to illustrate these disorders isn't easy. But one patient, Margaret, sticks out because she was the first patient that I took primary responsibility for treating as an out-patient in my first psychiatry job, and because she was unfortunately initially misdiagnosed with potentially dangerous results. She had gone to her GP complaining of pains in her stomach. He had sent her to the hospital to have tests to see if she had an ulcer. Though these were negative the surgeons had been asked to operate and she was being prepared to have part of her stomach removed—a partial gastrectomy. Luckily the GP asked for a second opinion, and she came to see me.

Soon in the interview it became clear that she was depressed and anxious and that the stomach ulcer was in fact 'butterflies' in her tummy. She had lost appetite and interest in life soon after her youngest son left home to go to university—leaving her bereft of her usual mothering role. I explained to her what I thought was going on, that she had depression and anxiety as a result of her last child moving out and recommended that she take a course of an antidepressant instead of the surgery. A few weeks later she was back to her old self. The depression had lifted and along with it the tummy symptoms. And she still had a fully intact stomach!

Depression is so common that it is perhaps unsurprising that so many different mental experiences are reported. Most are unpleasant and disturbing and some can be extremely distressing. Depressed people usually have negative thoughts. They frequently fear the worst for themselves and their families. Often, they feel that they have let other people down and worry about this. The ability of depression to distort thinking so that it becomes self-serving of the depression is one of the most insidious and damaging aspects of this psychiatric disorder. It explains why many people who suffer from depression do not seek treatment—they believe either that they are not ill, their thoughts are correct. Or worse, they can believe that they are so bad that they do not deserve help.

The content of depressive thinking is I believe clearly determined by the upbringing and education of the patient, i.e. is 'culturally bound.' Western Judaeo/Christian cultures have traditionally inculcated children with guilt when teaching social and other skills, and often refer to the *Bible* for examples of what will happen if behaviour falls short of the ideal. Particularly in faith-based schools it was commonly taught that being 'bad,' i.e. not conforming to adult biblical directives, will lead to damnation and a period of purgatory, or even eternity being spent with the Devil in Hell.

More modern attitudes to biblical teachings, and education, play down the actuality of such a place as Hell but the centuries over which these concepts have been incorporated into Western culture means that they are still very prominent as concepts. They can even override rational scientific thought. I clearly remember two American colleagues of mine who at a conference in Paris went to visit Notre Dame Cathedral. When I asked them over dinner how their day had gone they said 'Terribly.' The religious images contained in this grand Catholic church had, in both of them, brought back distressing memories of their schooling by Jesuits. There the threat of Hell and eternal punishment ('damnation') were the mainstay of discipline and formed the backbone of the teacher 'encouragement' for them to work hard. That such experiences in childhood can disrupt the minds of senior scientists 30 years later shows that the Jesuit adage 'Give me a boy by seven years and I will give you a believer for life' has some neurobiological underpinnings. One can't escape the memory content of one's formative years, particularly one in which the teachers chose to use threats and disturbing images as motivators.

In other cultures, depressive content will be consonant with local teachings, for example, being possessed by bad spirits or having a wicked spell put upon them by a witch doctor. As Western society evolves away from church-based ethical drives we can expect to see depression content also changing with sense of failure as an economic or emotional provider for one's family becoming more prominent than religion-based negative experiences. Such sense of being a failure is one of the main reasons so many depressed people commit suicide.

In recent year since the omnipresence of the computer depressed people sometimes speak of their brains as being locked into pointless loops of thinking ('ruminations'). When antidepressant treatments work then they can use the analogy of de-fragmenting or resetting their brain as if it was a computer hard drive.

In extreme cases depressive thinking can be so far removed from reality that it becomes delusional. For example, depressed patients with religious beliefs can develop the idea that they are working for the Devil and have committed unspeakable sins in his name. They may also believe the Devil is controlling their mind. It is not uncommon for such people with severe delusional depression to feel as if the Devil is sitting on their back. In extreme cases they may actually believe that they have become the Devil themselves.

One of the most distressing cases of depression I ever treated was in a Catholic priest who when depressed thought that instead of working for God he had all along been an agent of the Devil. This naturally caused him huge distress and led him to trying, against his religious beliefs, to commit suicide. When eventually we lifted him out of his depression with electro-compulsive therapy (ECT) he had no memory of this completely out-of-character belief system.

Depressive delusions can be held with such conviction that patients act on them. Many deaths of children are driven by depression in a parent with the associated belief that they will all suffer Hell on Earth so the parent kills both themself and the children to avoid the self-predicted suffering.

The delusional nature of depressive beliefs can be so profound that they reach the level of certainty even in experts such as psychiatrists who might be expected to have more insight than anyone that they are ill. One of the most famous and influential psychiatrists in the 1960s, the hugely qualified Professor Frank James Fish (1917–1968) of Liverpool University, whose specialism was psychological medicine, shot himself during an episode of depression after his colleagues minimised the severity of his condition and refused his request for ECT! Sadly, his case is not unique; many cases of depression are not treated appropriately leaving patients to act on their delusions and kill themselves.

Why depression leads to guilt feelings is a great mystery. We used to think that depressed thinking occurred because somehow the brain 'lost' its ability to have positive thoughts. This idea developed from the observations that loss events often are the cause of a depressive episode. Events shown to increase the risk of depression range through the most likely loss by death of a parent or partner or child (the most severe of all), through loss of a job or divorce and even to loss of a limb. This strong association between loss events and depression made psychiatrists think that we had somehow (in sympathy with the real loss) also lost the brain capacity to have positive thoughts. But recent brain research has shown exactly the opposite! The brain imaging work of the American neurologist Helen Mayberg, and confirmed by others since, has provided evidence that depression is a state of negative thinking that is imposed on the brain rather than being a loss of positive feelings. As William James (1842–1910) the US psychologist said of his depression, 'It is a positive and active anguish, a sort of psychical neuralgia wholly unknown to normal life.' We now know that there is a part of the brain that drives negative thinking that is overactive in depressed people and that most types of antidepressant treatments, from CBT to medicines to ECT, all reduce its activity.

The experience of the immovability of depressive thinking is well-captured by this quote from Thomas Carlyle (1795–1891), English man of letters, reflecting on his depression:

'It was one huge dead immeasurable steam-engine, rolling on in dead indifference to grind me limb from limb … having no hope.'

Many depressed patients talk of their mind being locked in repetitive 'tramlines' of thoughts from which they can't escape. We believe the efficacy of psychedelics such as psilocybin and ayahuasca to lift depression is due to these drugs disrupting these entrained thinking processes and allowing the person to see the world more normally.

Even if the brain can be set in a negative or pessimistic mode of thinking in depression perhaps through a deficit in serotonin, the content of depressive thoughts can't simply be generated by primary changes in neurotransmitter function. Their complex content with common themes must imply some prior learning and memory of moral and religious values that relate to guilt. These constructs then become personified and incorporated into the depressed persons sense of self by comparison with people or beliefs that have been learned of as being bad, such as the Devil or blackness.

Winston Churchill called his depression his 'Black Dog' which seemed to make sense of its subjective effects to those of his generation; 'dog days' being a common description of days of pointlessness and lack of achievement and black is often used as a description of the colour of depressive thinking, as per the so-called 'black thoughts' that lack the life and vitality that colours bring.

I think the best description of the mental experience of depression leading to suicide is in the book from which this chapter gets its title—*Darkness Visible: A Memoir of Madness* by William Stryon (see *Selected Bibliography*). This is an autobiography about his own depression by the prize-winning American author who is most famous for his book *Sophies' Choice*. He said this about depression which on one occasion was so bad it stopped him from collecting a literary award:

> 'The pain of severe depression is quite unimaginable to those who have not suffered it, and it kills in many instances because its anguish can no longer be borne. The prevention of many suicides will continue to be hindered until there is a general awareness of the nature of this pain. Through the healing process of time—and through medical intervention or hospitalization in many cases—most people survive depression, which may be its only blessing; but to the tragic legion who are compelled to destroy themselves there should be no more reproof attached than to the victims of terminal cancer.'

Sadly, many of his literary peers rejected Styron's descriptions of his mental suffering, and they savagely attacked him for admitting them—and even worse—taking medication. They spewed traditional 'intellectual's' misbelief that depression was a necessary element in the creative process that all artists experience. They argued that to complain about and to take medicines for depression was a form of moral cowardice. I hope his critics have all now read his book and apologised.

Where do bodily symptoms of depression come from?

How does the brain generate symptoms elsewhere in the body? The short answer is that we still don't know, but presumably it reflects the fact that the brain receives inputs from all the body and directs outputs to most of it. Even what we might assume to be basic reflex functions such as the secretion of stomach acid and production of urine can be directly influenced by brain activity. On top of this the brain releases hormones that can add to the neural influences, providing a more long-lived series of effects. In the case of the stomach the input is via the vagus nerve, that leaves the brain via the hole at the base of the skull and wanders down through the chest—where it sends out branches to control the rate the heart beats at—and then into the abdomen where it controls acid secretion in the stomach and the release of hormones from other parts of the upper gut.

Anxiety and depression increase the activity of the vagus nerve and this leads to symptoms that my patient Margaret (see earlier in this chapter) had — butterflies in her tummy and indigestion. Why this happens is not well-established but it may be part of a primitive defensive reaction to stress. The body trying to optimise the digestion of food so that the person's energy supplies can be maximised.

One theory why people become 'slowed-up' and 'lose drive and energy' in depression is that it's a form of hibernation. When a bear spends winter hibernating in a cave, it secretes hormones that make it enter a slowed-down metabolic state that allows it to keep alive for months without food or water. Some very depressed people enter a similar state, they slow-down, stop eating and drinking and their internal process also slows-up. Intestinal activity declines and they can become very constipated, and their heart rate also slows. This may be protective, a means by which people faced with insoluble stress can 'escape' for a while until it resolves. However, in extreme cases if untreated people with this extreme form of depression can become terminally starved and dehydrated and so die.

Preventing depression

In recent years it has become clear that antidepressants have an even greater role in preventing depression than in treating new episodes of it. They have a powerful protective effect to stop depressive episodes recurring. Antidepressants do this by increasing serotonin or noradrenaline but also, probably through increasing these neurotransmitters, elevate key brain hormones (such as brain derived neurotrophic factor (BDNF)) that keep nerve cells growing properly. They also increase resilience to stress by reducing stress hormones and modifying the brain's response to stress.

In people who have had several episodes of depression, keeping on the antidepressant is a powerful way of preventing a further relapse. In fact, this is one of the most powerful effects in modern medical therapeutics — around ten times more powerful than the ability of a statin to prevent a repeat heart attack!

We now take a very different attitude to depression than we did 30 years ago treating it as a chronic relapsing disorder, like epilepsy, rather than as a single sporadic disorder such as a broken leg or bout of pneumonia.

A good example of this is another patient of mine—Howard. He was a thoughtful, gentle 30-year-old who had lost his job as a teacher a year previously because he had been unable to work on account of his depressions. He'd had seven of these bouts in the past five years and each had been successfully treated by his GP with antidepressants. However, each time after his mood had lifted the GP assumed he was 'cured' and stopped the antidepressant. Within months he had relapsed and so was unable to work for several months till the GP prescribed another course of antidepressant and these started working.

The cycle was then repeated until on the seventh episode the school dismissed him on the grounds of repeated ill-health, so adding to his stress and depression. If only he had been kept on his medicine for a few years he might still be working today!

Current evidence suggests that even a single episode of depression makes people much more vulnerable to future episodes. In one series of 50 patients with a first attack of depression who were followed up for 25 years, all but one (98 per cent) had had a second episode of depression in this period. This suggests that in most cases depression will recur. The leading explanation for this vulnerability to repeat episodes is the idea of a 'scar' being left in the brain after the first episode that can be opened-up by further stress, life events and medical illnesses. Although antidepressants may not heal the scar, they can protect it from stress and other causes of depression as a form of 'chemical sticking plaster,' but this is lost if the antidepressant is stopped. We therefore recommend for people who have had three or more depressive episodes already that long-term treatment with antidepressants should be seriously considered.

An interesting comparison is with epilepsy (*Chapter 13*) where the persistence of the scar can be objectively measured by EEG or brain imaging. The scar contains an excess of neurons that excites the brain so making repeat seizures more likely. Here the default position is that anti-epilepsy drugs are used for years and are only stopped following a conscious agreement between patient and doctor. Similarly, we no longer ask how long we should treat a patient with depression but, rather, when have they been well enough for long enough that it might be an appropriate time to stop.

The decision to stop an antidepressant is a vital one that needs to be made with the fully-informed consent of the patient and ideally key family members too. Every time someone becomes depressed there is a small but real risk (around five-to-ten per cent) that they will fail to recover. Thus, the more often someone becomes depressed the more likely it is that they will experience non-response.

I have seen many of my patients—often the doctors amongst them—decide that they can stop their treatment when well on the assumption that even if they relapse a reinstatement of their antidepressant will quickly restore their mood. But on occasions this doesn't happen, the new episode of depression is in some as yet unknown way different to the old one. It has become resistant to the old medicine, much to the chagrin of the patient, and the psychiatrist who then has to struggle to find another medicine that works.

Serotonin seems critical in maintaining wellness when people have recovered from depression. In a landmark study of the brain chemistry of depression relapse the group of Dennis Charney at Yale University, USA in the 1990s showed that for depressed patients who have recovered on serotonin-enhancing antidepressants, e.g. SSRIs, depletion of serotonin led to a relapse over just a few hours. In one patient of theirs in this study the relapse resulted in the Devil returning to control her thoughts like he had done before treatment. Reassuringly for the investigators, the Devil soon disappeared once the serotonin levels in her brain were restored by giving a high protein meal that quickly restored tryptophan to the brain. The fact that the same content of thoughts can return in another episode of depression just a few hours after reducing serotonin in the brain tells us that these thoughts are probably always there—they haven't gone away despite the mood having lifted.

From this finding the idea has developed that depression is always lurking in the brain; so that patients who have had one episode of depression are always more vulnerable to another episode than those of us who have never been depressed. We now believe that depressive and anxious thoughts and mood are normally kept at bay by positive thoughts or by some other form of top-down cortical control (probably from the prefrontal cortex) that suppresses the subcortical brain regions such as the limbic system that drive depressive thinking.

We believe that the protective effect of serotonin in depression is mediated through the activation of a subtype of serotonin receptor—the 5-HT1A receptor—in the limbic system. This provides resilience and buffers the person against the strains and stresses of life that tend to lead to depression. But to do this the antidepressant medicines have to be taken daily. Recently we and others have shown that a single treatment with the psychedelic drug psilocybin can also have an antidepressant effect. Psilocybin and other psychedelics work through stimulation of the 5-HT2A receptor which is largely located in the cerebral cortex. The effects of just a single psilocybin treatment can last for many months which suggests that they are mediated through a different process to that of the SSRIs. Our current theory is that during the psilocybin-induced psychedelic trip, the repetitive negative thinking that is so characteristic of depression is fundamentally disrupted. This means that for the first time in months or years the depressed person can experience a depression-free period.

It may be that this insight allows them to maintain a more positive mental attitude once the drug effect has worn off. Perhaps more likely is that the transient disruption to the ongoing ruminative brain processes helps to stop these maladaptive brain processes from re-forming. Either, or even both of, these processes, could explain why many of our patients reported that as a result of the psilocybin treatment they had, for the first time, understood and been able to overcome their depression.

The fact that some of our patients stayed depression-free for months supports the idea that the effects of psilocybin on depression are profoundly different from those of SSRIs. Psilocybin seems to allow patients to overcome their depression rather than just suppress it as the SSRIs do. But after the immediate benefit from psilocybin that we saw in almost all our patients, within a few weeks or months about half found that their depression was beginning to recur. This suggests that the underlying propensity to depression, whether genetic or environmental, was still present and pushing them into the low mood. It may be that psychedelic treatment for depression is something that should be administered on a regular basis, maybe two or three times a year, to keep people in the depression-free state.

CHAPTER 14

Why Worry? Fear and Anxiety Disorders

In many ways anxiety (which I touched on in *Chapter 13*) is the opposite of depression—the body speeds up—the heart races—breathing rates increase—muscles tighten-up—the mind becomes alert and focused. This is the classic 'fight or flight' reaction that prepares animals for the necessary bodily changes when threatened. Energy availability is increased to provide for more vigorous muscle activity and the heart and breathing speed up to get more oxygen to the muscles. The brain is focused on the threat to the detriment of wider inputs. This all makes sense when there really is a physical threat—and presumably these reactions were valuable when early humans were fighting for survival against wild animals or hostile tribes. They are still necessary today when fighting in war or against an assailant but when they occur without there being a physical threat they are very unsettling.

The mental arousal is felt as anxiety and the pounding heart and churning lungs as a panic. Mental focus is altered, and this can lead to a total preoccupation with fearful thoughts—worries—or can be on specific feared things such as spiders or other phobic objects. Persistent mental over-arousal or anxiety leads to headaches as the facial muscles are in a state of over-constriction.

Thinking processes and more especially thought content in anxiety disorders are quite different to that in depression (*Chapter 13*). The content is worrying or in more extreme cases fearful. This is why we tend now to divide up anxiety disorders into two groups—'worry disorders' and 'fear disorders.' The most common worry disorder is called generalised anxiety disorder or GAD. People with GAD are continually concerned about things going wrong in the future. They see potential threats in everything around them. Every phone call could mean bad news. Every official brown envelope through the door is a police charge. Every twitch under their skin is a sign of cancer, etc. In the latter case this can develop into a condition we call health anxiety where people seek repeated medical assessments to prove they are not ill (hypochondriasis).

Fear disorders range from simple phobias—e.g. fear of spiders and heights through panic and social anxiety disorders to PTSD. The brain processes, neurotransmitters and fear circuits underpinning these are described in *Chapters 2* and *8*. At the simplest level the fear response leads to avoidance of the threat stimulus (e.g. a spider) plus attentional monitoring of the threat to ensure if it moves the person stays well away. The fear circuit is inborn and explains why with some fears—e.g. of heights—even young children won't crawl over a visual cliff (a glass plate over a gap in the floor). But for most fears the linking of the object to an external stimulus requires learning—usually from parents.

Baby monkeys need to be taught to be fearful of snakes by their mothers and this acquired fear requires glutamate neurotransmitter-induced learning in the amygdala. Similarly in humans, children mimic the fear their parents or peers have of spiders and mice. When mum screams at a mouse and jumps up on a chair to escape children tend to get scared and follow suit. The behaviour perpetuates through the generations. But there is likely some evolutionary brain predisposition to acquiring fears of animals that are potentially harmful, that makes these phobias so rapidly acquired. In the same way as baby birds have an innate fear of the shape of hawks.

Sometimes the fear circuit can suddenly activate for no reason. This is rather like an epilepsy seizure but in a different brain circuit, the fear rather than motor pathways. These attacks are called 'panic attacks' and are very distressing to the person experiencing them. They feel frightened and shaky, feel their heart beating fast, their breathing accelerated (they feel it's difficult to get enough air) and often they feel cold and light-headed. Sometimes they may faint. If this occurs a lot and impairs the person's life then they have a condition called 'panic disorder.'

Because these panic attacks are so powerfully unpleasant and aversive, people remember them vividly and so avoid the memory of them by not going back to where they happened, which also helps to avoid future attacks. This avoidance leads to the condition of agoraphobia where people may refuse to go into the place where the panic happened, e.g. a supermarket, or to where they feel an attack might occur and from which escape might be difficult, e.g.

on a train or bus. They then avoid all supermarkets or public transport in case other attacks occur in such places.

You may ask, 'Why do panic attacks tend to occur in supermarkets?' The answer is that they are social places and agoraphobia means 'fear of the market-place.' Anxiety is provoked by the presence of other people and by not having access to a safe refuge. The marketplace — or now the supermarket — is large, noisy and busy with no obvious safe place to escape to. Sensory stimulation like the bright lights and noise in supermarkets also tend to excite the brain and provoke anxiety (in the same way they can provoke seizures in people with some forms of epilepsy). This is why some people with panic disorders find that dark glasses or polarising ones reduce their risk of an attack. In severe cases the agoraphobia can be so powerful that the person refuses even to go out of the house, putting a huge burden on their family.

During a panic attack the person feels as if they are ill or even dying. This leads them to seek help and they often call for an ambulance or go to the emergency room thinking they are having a heart attack or asthma attack. Inevitably a physical examination reveals no medical problem and the patient is reassured and sent home.

Sometimes expensive medical tests are conducted to prove there is no under-lying pathology and this leads to considerable waste of National Health Service (NHS) resources. But the reassurance doesn't work — the panic attacks persist because the brain fear circuit is still over-reactive. Dampening down this circuit can be done using antidepressant medicines especially the SSRIs that calm this circuit in the same way as they calm the depression circuit.

Alternatively, cognitive behaviour therapy (CBT) can be used. This works by getting the patient to understand that the cognitions that accompany a panic attack — the fear that one might be ill — are false beliefs. The therapist then gets the patient to develop these thoughts and helps them to gather evidence for the veracity or falsehood of each. They can then use this evidence and reason to sup-press the incorrect thinking. Thinking in people with panic disorder frequently exaggerates the medical impact of the symptoms, often in a catastrophic way. For example, a patient may experience a slight change in heart rate and inter-pret this as that they might be having a heart attack. This thought then leads to them becoming very anxious and even panicky and often seeking medical help.

The behavioural element involves what is called exposure therapy—the person is encouraged to re-visit the place where the panics happened in a gradual fashion, and often with someone there to support them. They spend longer and longer in the situation and gradually learn that the fear can be controlled, and they don't succumb to the presumed underlying medical illness. Over time the fear itself starts to disappear; a process called 'extinction.'

We came across PTSD in *Chapter 2* as a brain (and bodily) response to life-threatening stress. The memory of the fear response re-emerges suddenly often overwhelming the person's ability to behave normally. The thought content of PTSD is subtly different from that of panic attack. In panic the person thinks that the bodily symptoms mean that they might be ill or even dying, but in PTSD they know that they are at risk of dying—because they have previously been in such a situation. This is why people with PTSD who have attacks in states of reduced consciousness such as sleep can fight back like they did during the original trauma, often with disastrous effects on bed partners.

Social anxiety is almost the defining human condition. Young children are frightened of strangers and for most of us some of this anxiety persists into adult life. That's why the first thing served at parties is alcohol because it dampens down the anxiety that we all feel in public situations, especially with people we don't know. For some people this is so severe that they can't socialise, and, if they try to, they blush and may panic and run away, which then adds more stress the next time they try.

The cognitions of social anxiety are centred on what other people are thinking about the sufferer—thoughts like, 'I am making a fool of myself' serve to compound the anxiety and impair the ability to talk sensibly, so the anxiety becomes self-reinforcing. Many young men with social anxiety turn to alcohol to deal with it and can end up alcoholics as a result. In fact, social anxiety disorder is the commonest cause of alcohol dependence in young men. Luckily, it can be rectified either by SSRIs or by specialised CBT.

One special example of extreme social anxiety is the fear of public speaking. Some people say they are more fearful of this than dying. It is well-known that young men will break off an engagement to be married because that event requires a public speech. I have seen three such cases in my clinical career and am pleased to say that each one responded well to an SSRI, so the ceremony went ahead to the relief of everyone.

CHAPTER 15

Delusional? Schizophrenia and Mania

S chizophrenia and mania are highly damaging psychiatric disorders with very negative consequences to those who suffer from them, their families and friends. They often start in adolescence; schizophrenia often with subtle alterations in behaviour in the early-teens that, at around 20 years-of-age can develop into frank hallucinations and delusions. Mania onset is often much more sudden as a result of stress, or sometimes drug use.

Schizophrenia

Schizophrenia to the psychiatrist is one of the most challenging disorders to treat as we have a very limited range of medicines and a significant proportion of patients do not respond well to these. To the neuroscientist schizophrenia is a fascinating condition that asks many questions about how the brain works and how consciousness becomes disordered. The fact that schizophrenia is seen in about one per cent of all different population groups worldwide tells us it is not simply socially-determined. But it is clear that social stress can make schizophrenia worse and outcomes for city-based patients more so than for those living in the more sheltered world of the countryside. Schizophrenia is also strongly genetic but very many different genes are involved so it seems likely that there are, equally, many different forms of schizophrenia.

The patient's changes in thinking in schizophrenia are diagnostic. There are three main changes, and they may have only one or several of them. Most well-known are delusions, which are false beliefs that are often firmly-held and unshakable even when the person is confronted by contradictory evidence.

Delusions

Delusions are commonly called 'paranoia' and largely feature concerns about threats to the person. Examples include a belief that one is being talked about or spied upon. Often altered perceptions, particularly of smell, are taken as evidence of this interference and sufferers will confront their neighbours with complaints that they are putting radio waves through the wall or poison gas under the door to harm them. The perplexed denial of the neighbours may lead to angry exchanges and even physical altercations. In extreme cases the paranoid person may attack and even kill the presumed perpetrator.

If they can do so, paranoid people may move to escape the person they believe is victimising them. But, usually, a new delusion develops in the new environment; one patient of mine even changed continents but the paranoid ideas re-emerged. Paranoid delusions are ideas that have abnormal salience (meaning) to the patient. We have probably all experienced a sense that someone is talking about us behind our back. When this moves from a feeling that can easily be rationalised away to become an unshakeable belief it becomes a delusion.

Often people who go on to develop schizophrenia experience a period during which they feel that something is 'not right' and that things are going on that have meaning or relevance to them. This can last for weeks or even months but then commonly this feeling either disappears or 'crystalises' into a sense of certainty, which we call a delusional belief. These delusions can be simple in content, e.g. that the neighbours are listening to them, or can become quite complicated with governments and even extra-terrestrial beings getting woven into complex paranoid stories of impending world domination.

The process through which the brain attaches increased meaning of events appears to be driven by alterations in dopamine function. We know that drugs that release dopamine, e.g. cocaine can lead to paranoid ideas that build-up over the course of a weekend binge on this drug. Also drugs that block dopamine receptors are the mainstay of treatment for paranoid schizophrenia. Dopamine is thought to determine the salience of events, with more dopamine leading to more salience. The crystallisation process probably involves higher centres in the cortex.

Mania

Delusions in mania are usually quite different from those in schizophrenia, being positive rather than threatening or critical. People experiencing a manic episode may begin to believe that they have special abilities and that they are more clever and more creative than other people. In more extreme cases they may believe they have special powers and are in touch with God—or even that they are Jesus Christ, Buddha, Mohammed or some other deity reincarnated.

Manic delusions differ from those of schizophrenia in terms of the mood component—manic ones being associated with enhanced mood whereas in schizophrenia they are usually negative and hostile. These states also differ, in that manic patients are much more likely to act on their delusions—they can fully lose insight. If a manic person believes they are, say Jesus, they usually start dressing in gowns and blessing people. In schizophrenia delusions are less likely to be acted out, suggesting a degree of insight—or at least uncertainty—may still exist.

As with schizophrenic delusions these manic delusions respond well to treatment with dopamine-blocking drugs, which suggests that this neurotransmitter has some role in their genesis. In fact, the consciousness changes in mania are more obviously linked to dopamine than are those found in schizophrenia. They replicate the feelings of increased energy, drive, self-confidence and sexuality, plus the reduced need for sleep that are found with dopamine-releasing stimulants such as cocaine and crystal meth.

Other aspects of altered consciousness in schizophrenia

The two other key altered consciousness elements of schizophrenia are hallucinations and thought disorder.

Hallucinations

Hallucinations are common in schizophrenia and are usually auditory in nature. They often start as unintelligible sounds for which the person can't locate a source. Then they progress to simple words such as the calling of the person's name. As the illness progresses then the voices take on a more persistent nature, initially one voice (usually the same 'person') making a running commentary of the patient's actions or thoughts. These take the form of negative comments such as:

'Why is he going to the shops, he hasn't got any money?'

Or

'Don't talk to your mother today.'

However, in some cases the content can be more supportive and positive.

Some socially-isolated people with schizophrenia, for whom the voices may be the only human voices they encounter with any regularity, may come to feel them as being 'friends.'

In the worst cases, several different 'persons' voices may be heard, often engaging in a critical and hostile dialogue about the patient. These are sometimes the voices of parents or other significant individuals in the person's life or are from 'unknown people.' They may be of either gender and sometimes one is male and another female. As well as criticising the person's behaviour, feelings and attitudes they may try to make the sufferer do things against their will—so called 'made' feelings. In addition to being distressing to the person who has to resist these internal instructions, if they can't resist then they can be compelled to act on them. These 'made actions' can have disastrous consequences as the voices can direct them to harm other people, set fire to property and even commit suicide.

A critical running commentary on one's life and behaviour is, naturally, quite distressing even if the person with schizophrenia realises that the voices are from inside their own head. It's worse when they try to locate the source of them as external to their body. They may look for loudspeakers in the furniture or even outside the house. When they can't locate these, then they often develop delusional ideas such as that they have had transmitters implanted into their ears or teeth to relay the voices.

The origins of the voices are obviously from inside the head and most likely the brain (as opposed to the hearing apparatus of the ear). Psychoanalysts saw them as reflecting the patient's own thoughts spoken aloud though in a different voice. As we saw in *Chapter 7* recent neuroimaging studies show this to have some validity. We now believe voices occur because of a failure of the inner brain mechanisms that inform the auditory cortex that speech is being developed in the language cortex.

Thought disorder

The other feature of schizophrenia in this section is thought disorder, where ideas and thinking get mixed up or produced somewhat out of sequence or logic. The usual logical thread of consciousness is disrupted so a mixture of different elements or themes is produced. Irregular jumps in logical connections occur and this is called 'knights move thinking' after the chess piece that can move diagonally, left or right, as well as backwards and forwards. In severe cases language can become garbled and unintelligible to the listener. Thought disorder occurs because the normal integrative processes of control from the frontal cortex become disturbed.

Different combinations

People with schizophrenia may show one or more of these three elements of altered consciousness. Often paranoid ideas exist in isolation, and sufferers can live relatively normal lives despite their delusions. This coupled with the fact that paranoid ideas often develop later in life suggests simple delusional schizophrenia is a different syndrome to those disorders that start in teenage years with complex delusions thought disorder and hallucinations. Brain imaging studies have shown that these different elements of schizophrenia emerge from different regions of the brain and probably represent dysfunction in different functional circuits.

CHAPTER 16

Repetition, Obsession and Compulsion

OCD is shorthand for 'obsessive-compulsive disorder.' This is a set of mental activities and behaviours characterised by repetitive actions or thoughts. The person knows they are unnecessary, pointless, and even damaging, but they are compelled to do them because, if they don't, then they get very anxious. Some people have obsessive behaviours and others obsessive repetitive thoughts, and some both of these.

The mental content of obsessions typically centres around germs and contamination and the fear of illnesses developing from them. These thoughts can lead patients to wash their hands repeatedly to the point where their skin becomes raw and inflamed. In extreme cases they may wash ten-to-20 times after a single use of the toilet. In extreme cases they may even resort to using bleach to ensure skin sterility with even more damaging consequences to their body.

To minimise contact with 'germs' some patients will limit access to their house and even keep a special 'clean room' in it that only they are allowed to use. The major fears of contamination are from viruses on other peoples' hands and germs from dog faeces. To protect themselves from these they may wear gloves to open their mail or read a newspaper as these have been handled by strangers, who might be 'unclean.' Some repeatedly clean their homes — vacuuming and dusting several times a day.

Another common obsession is the fear of stepping on the gaps between paving stones, well demonstrated by Jack Nicholson in the film 'As Good as it Gets.' This is a ritual that often starts with a 'silly' thought (incorporated in many societal myths) that harm will come if one steps on a gap. Then as the person gets more practised in avoiding them the behaviour becomes a habit that like all other habits is hard to break.

The English writer Dr Samuel Johnson had a range of these. He had a special ritual when passing through doors, counting the steps into them, and then often twirling around with a jump when he passed through. Also, to the great concern of his associates, when drinking tea, he would extend the arm holding the cup in the four directions of the compass before supping it.

Obsessive thinking takes different forms. Some people need to count a certain number of times before they do anything. This may turn into 'checking behaviour' when they have to check every switch and water tap in their house that number of times before they can leave. Others have to repeat obscene or religious thoughts a certain number of times. They feel compelled to repeatedly enact this ritual even though they know it is not necessary and in some cases, particularly where there is obscene content, it can be highly distressing.

Usually, people with OCD know that their behaviour is unnecessary and pointless, i.e. they have insight and understand that it's their brain, not their mind, making them do it. The motivation for OCD is therefore not like in schizophrenia where actions are felt as being put into the brain. Often patients with OCD resist doing the action, but the longer they resist the greater the urge or compulsion to do it. Eventually this urge and the rising level of anxiety that accompanies it leads to their giving in to it and completing the behaviour. They then experience a surge of pleasurable relief that terminates their anxiety and allows them to lead a normal life until the next bout, which can be within a few hours to several days.

How does this strange behaviour start? Often OCD begins quite innocuously—probably we have all had a trivial thought, such as that the oven might be left on, and so have checked that it's not. Finding we were right and that it was switched off is reassuringly pleasurable. In some people the relief this sense of certainty produces leads to them repeating the behaviour. In people with OCD there is a gradual escalation in the number of times the checking is perpetuated and so the OCD develops.

The fact that obsessions about cleanliness are most common in women straight after childbirth suggests that they reflect an exaggerated natural biological nurturing process. Intense cleaning can be seen as an extreme form of normal grooming behaviour that may be accentuated by the hormonal changes post childbirth. There is also a learning component and obsessions can run in families as children model on their parents. There is also evidence of altered brain circuits relating to decision-making and impulsivity in patients with OCD and in near family relatives.

An alternative explanation is that the motoric and other thought processes are simply overlearned behaviours, aka habits—like nail-biting and hair-twisting. This has biological credibility as brain imaging studies have shown that people with OCD have over-activity in a brain circuit that includes parts of the basal ganglia, a brain region that regulates movements. For this reason, OCD can be considered a disorder of excessive repetitive actions or habits.

The discovery of the brain circuit perpetuating OCD is now leading to attempts to dampen this by using neurosurgical brain stimulation approaches. This approach is widely used to reduce abnormal movements in people with Parkinson's disease and is now being tested in people with OCD in specialist neurosurgery centres.

Compulsive thinking is harder to explain but probably reflects the innate tendency of brains to think and compute. Some forms of repetitive thinking may be reassuring in the same way that repeated skin stroking can be calming to children and as massage in adults. Repeated chanting can be relaxing because it switches off the thinking centres of the brain. Some religious orders encourage this form of repetition in either prayer or signing to facilitate engagement with God. Repetition is somehow reassuring, perhaps because it fits with one of the of the key aspects of how the brain works.

We saw in *Chapter 5* that the brain predicts and assumes stability in the environment and is especially activated by change. OCD patients want security and stability in their environment and their brain is trying to get them this, but at the cost of failing in other ways.

CHAPTER 17

From Pleasure to Pain? Addiction

Although most people tend to think of addiction as being a disorder driven by seeking pleasure from drugs it has another side—that of the pain of being unable to stop using them. When addiction becomes an entrenched behaviour it bears many similarities with OCD-type compulsive behaviours (*Chapter 16*), but one that focuses on either alcohol/drugs or behaviours such as gambling or internet use. The addict doesn't want to keep using but the drives in their brain override their mind's capacity (their willpower) to prevent them continuing with the behaviour.

It is a myth that most drug addicts enjoy taking drugs. Perhaps at the beginning some do, but over time as the behaviour becomes more and more entrenched, this effect is lost and the drug use becomes habitual and even despised by the user; but they can't stop. As author Edgar Alan Poe wrote so poignantly in a letter in the last years of his life:

> 'I have absolutely no pleasure in the stimulants in which I sometimes so madly indulge. It has not been in the pursuit of pleasure that I have periled life and reputation and reason. It has been the desperate attempt to escape from torturing memories, from a sense of insupportable loneliness and a dread of some strange impending doom.'

The initiation of these behaviours is usually benign and is often in a social setting, though in the case of alcohol it may be to deal with problems such as anxiety and stress. Over time, in a proportion of people the drug/behaviour becomes more important to the person, they begin to become dependent on it and engage in it more to the exclusion of social activities. At some point they can't stop, which is when we say they are addicted. In this phase the addict pursues a path of activities that they know is damaging them psychologically, financially, socially and in terms of family life.

Like people with OCD, addicts usually resist the urge to continue to engage in these behaviours but then give in as the drive to use (craving) overwhelms their ability to control them. As in the case of OCD, addicts get a great relief when they submit to the urge to use (the word 'craving' comes from the Latin for cowardly and this reflects the long-held view by the general public that addicts lack the moral fibre or will to overcome their desires). Also like with people with OCD the addict often then feels bad about having given in to their cravings and can feel remorseful or even depressed about this (usually repeated) failure of theirs.

Where drug addiction differs from OCD is that the brain processes on which drugs act are the very ones that regulate these behaviours. So, for example stimulants like cocaine and methamphetamine turn on the brain's dopamine system so enhancing drive and energy and producing long-lasting adaptive changes that work to perpetuate use of these drugs. Alcohol does the same but to a lesser extent. However it also affects the part of the brain that is necessary to control these drives (the pre-frontal cortex (PFC)) and so reduces 'top down' control of behaviour.

Most of us will know someone (even perhaps ourselves) who starts drinking with the genuine intention of only 'having a couple of drinks' but when the alcohol begins to turn-off their frontal lobes they seem to change their personality and lose self-control, going on a binge or even worse getting into fights, etc.

Heroin and other opioids act predominantly on the higher brain centres taking the person to a place so much 'better' than their current one so that they desire to go there again-and-again. If they don't have the opioid the craving for it can be so pronounced that they will steal from friends and family, prostitute themselves or commit impulsive crimes to get money for it.

The more a drug or behaviour is engaged in, the greater the likelihood of withdrawal setting in when it is stopped. Withdrawal can be very unpleasant (and in the case of alcohol life-threatening) and so the fear of this becomes a powerful motivation for continuing the addictive behaviour. In the case of heroin, we have drugs like buprenorphine and methadone that can prevent withdrawal and remove this fear. Currently, in some countries, baclofen and sodium oxybate are being used for the same purposes for alcohol dependence. The problem is that they have to be used continually, which means that the person becomes dependent on the substitute drug rather than on the primary addictive one.

Despite this drawback such substitutes are preferable for several reasons. They are free as medicines — so the addict doesn't need to commit crime to buy drugs anymore. They are safer than the original drug. For example, in the case of using buprenorphine for heroin addiction the risk of dying from over-dose is very much lower. And they are provided as medicines so are given in a standard dose and in a pure form, quite different from the very uncertain nature of street drugs, and so are much safer.

These substitute drug approaches have been hugely successful in reducing deaths and other harms (e.g. from HIV due to the use of unsterile needles, etc.) from opioid addiction, and to a lesser extent in some countries, reducing alcohol-related deaths. But they are still dependence-producing and many patients want to come off them. Also, despite several decades of research, there are no substitute treatments for cocaine and other stimulant addiction.

Currently, there are few medical options to help addicts 'stay clean/dry' once they have undergone withdrawal. For opioid addiction we can use drugs that block the opioid receptor such as naltrexone. These work well if taken but once they are stopped then a day later the person is vulnerable again. For this reason, longer-acting depot injections (i.e. of medication which releases slowly to permit less frequent administration) are being developed that might give protection for a month or more. As was mentioned in *Chapter 6*, because part of the effect of overdosing on alcohol is through the release of endorphins, opioid receptor antagonists such as nalmefene and naltrexone can be used to help alcoholics stay sober or reduce drinking.

This is a major medical need since over three quarters of all people who stop using and become 'clean' from their addiction relapse within a year. Psychedelic drugs such as psilocybin offer a new approach to addiction. In the current era there have been studies of just a few of doses of psilocybin as therapy, for people with tobacco and alcohol addiction, with great success. For example, Matt Johnson at Johns Hopkins University, USA has found that three psilocybin treatments over six months resulted in three-quarters of smokers quitting for good—by far the best result of any anti-smoking treatment ever. Similarly, Michael Bogenschutz at the University of New Mexico found a profound reduction in alcohol intake after just one psilocybin session.

These findings are not as surprising as they might seem at first sight. We know from research done in the 1950s and 1960s with a more powerful psychedelic—LSD—that it could lead to profound reductions in alcohol drinking. The banning of these drugs in the 1960s once they were used outside of medicine, stopped all associated research for nearly 50 years to the great detriment of patients with addictions. Luckily, it is making a resurgence and we hope that trials in other addictions such as opioids and stimulants will start soon.

How do psychedelics stop addiction is a key question. From our brain imaging research, we see that these drugs disrupt the brain circuits that contain and drive the habitual thinking processes that lock the addict into their behaviour. One of Matt Johnson's patients said of their relationship to tobacco after their psilocybin treatment, 'It no longer featured in my life.' The psilocybin trip seemed to have erased the habitual tramline thinking about tobacco that dependence on it produces.

CHAPTER 18

Brain and Mind or Brain-v-Mind?

In Part 2 of this book we have seen that the human mind can experience many different forms of consciousness and thought processes. Some of these are part of relatively rare and severe neurological and psychiatric disorders but others, such as nightmares and dreams are experienced by almost everyone. Each of these different forms of consciousness tell us something about the function of the brain and opens-up as yet unanswered questions about how they are produced and what they mean to the person experiencing them. They raise important challenges to neuroscience since a full understanding of how the brain works must be able to account for their origins and their content.

From my perspective as a psychiatrist, the most challenging and intriguing aspects of these altered workings of the mind is both why they occur, which parts of the brain mediates them, and why do some of them persist despite the person not wanting or even resisting them?

Most neuroscientists agree that the mind is an emergent property of the brain, without the brain there is no mind. But the fact that the brain processes and thought content in conditions such as OCD, addiction and schizophrenia are disliked and opposed in the minds of the people suffering them tells us something very important — there can be a conflict between brain and mind. Or perhaps it's between mind and mind — the classic split mind concept for which the term schizophrenia was coined. The size and complexity of the human brain means it is perfectly plausible that different forms of mind could emerge in the same person just as multiple personalities can exist in some people.

We have all had the experience of conflict between the brain and mind. There will be many examples of us wanting something but having to resist because of personal, social or other constraints. The human brain, especially after a few years of training in childhood is particularly good at top down cognitive or volitional control of drives and urges, so usually the consciousness volitional mind wins out. But the brain is also a remarkable learning machine which is why some learnt behaviours such as those in OCD and addiction can come to dominate over the volitional mind. Those learnt behaviours have the same basis as simple motor habits but are harder to suppress because they have significant emotional overlay. The reason people continue with them is because they are driven both by habit and desire, whereas wanting to stop them is just a desire.

Conflicts between brain and mind are seen in most of the conditions I have discussed. We often desire to sleep but our brain keeps us awake. People with schizophrenia want to get rid of the voices but their brain keeps them recurring. People with worry know there is no point to it, but their brain can't stop the habitual thoughts.

It's really only in depression and mania that abnormal thinking becomes congruent with the person's mind and that's what makes them such devastating disorders. Depressed people come to believe their thinking that they are bad and worthless and so retreat from help, sometimes to the point of suicide. Manic episodes are the opposite in that the thought content is clearly over-positive, yet the person believes and acts on those thoughts. Treatments for these disorders that just rely on re-organizing thinking such as CBT fail because of this loss of insight into the need to change the patient's thought content.

Some people with bipolar disorder can switch between depression and mania, sometimes in quick succession, even overnight. This suggests that there must be some kind of mood generator, or regulator, in the brain that directs whether thought contents are positive or negative. Locating this is an important target for psychiatry as it might lead to new treatments. As yet, all we can say is that the neurotransmitter serotonin seems to be involved in protecting against depression whereas dopamine seems to promote mania.

Selected Bibliography

Alexander, Eben (2012 reprint), *Proof of Heaven: A Neurosurgeon's Journey into the Afterlife*, Piatkus.

Browning, Christopher (1992), *Ordinary Men: Reserve Police Battalion 101 and the Final Solution in Poland*, HarperCollins.

Doble A, Martin I L and Nutt D J (2004), *Calming the Brain: Benzodiazepines and Related Drugs from Laboratory to Clinic*, Martin Dunitz Ltd.

Fish, Frank (1974 reprint), *Fish's Clinical Psychopathology*, John Wright & Sons.

Grey Walter, William (1953), *The Living Brain*, Gerald Duckworth & Co.

Haddad, Peter and Nutt, David (2020), *Seminars in Clinical Psychopharmacology*, Cambridge University Press.

Huxley, Alduous (1952), *The Devils of Loudon*, Harper & Brothers.

Huxley, Alduous (1959), *The Doors of Perception: And Heaven and Hell*, Penguin.

Iversen, Leslie, Iversen, Susan, Bloom, Floyd and Roth, Robert (2009), *Introduction to Neuropharmacology*, Blackwells.

James, William (1902), *The Varieties of Religious Experience*, Longmans Green & Co.

Jaspers, Karl (1963 translation), *General Psychopathology*, Manchester University Press.

Kandel, Eric, Koester, John, Mack, Sarah and Siegelbaum, Steven (2021), *Principles of Neural Science*, Blackwells.

Kennedy, Sidney, Lam, Raymond, Nutt, David and Thase, Michael (2017), *Treating Depression Effectively*, Informa.

Marks, Isaac (1987), *Fears Phobias and Rituals*, Oxford University Press.

Nutt, David (2019), *Drugs: Without the Hot Air*, edn. 2, UIT Press.

Nutt, David (2020), *Drink?*, Yellow Kite.

Nutt, David (2020), *Nutt Uncut*, Waterside Press.

Nutt, David, Stein, Murray and Zohar, Jossi (2006), *Post traumatic Stress Disorder: Diagnosis, Management and Treatment*, edn. 2, Taylor & Francis.

Nutt, David, Robbins, Trevor, Stimson, Gerald, Ince, Martin and Jackson, Martin (2007). *Drugs and the Future*, Academic Press.

Nutt, David and Nestor, Liam (2017), *Substance Abuse*, edn. 2, Oxford University Press.

O'Keane, Veronica (2021), *The Rag and Bone Shop*, Penguin.

Proust, Marcel (1934), *Remembrance of Things Past*, Random House (originally published as *À La Recherche du Temps Perdu* in seven parts between 1913 and 1927).

Rolls, Edmund (2016), *Cerebral Cortex: Principles of Operation*, Oxford Centre for Computational Neuroscience.

Sacks, Oliver (1973), *Awakenings,* Gerald Duckworth & Co.

Stetka, Bruce (2021), *A History of the Human Brain*, Timber Press.

Stryon, William (1990), *Darkness Visible: A
Memoir of Madness,* Random House.

Van der Kolk, Bessel (2015), *The Body Keeps the Score,* Penguin.

Walker, Mathew (2018), *Why We Sleep*, Penguin.

Wilson, Sue and Nutt David (2013), *Sleep
Disorders,* Oxford Psychiatry Library.

Wolpert, Lewis (2006), *Malignant Sadness: The
Anatomy of Depression,* edn.3, Faber & Faber.

Young, J Z (1978), *Programmes of the Brain*, Oxford University Press.

Young, Susan, et al (2018), 'Identification and treatment of
offenders with attention-deficit/hyperactivity disorder in the
prison population: a practical approach based upon expert
consensus,' September 4, *BMC Psychiatry*: www.researchgate.net/
publication/51637525_ADHD_and_offenders (accessed 21 June 2021).

Index

Nutt Uncut

David Nutt

Foreword Ilana B Crome

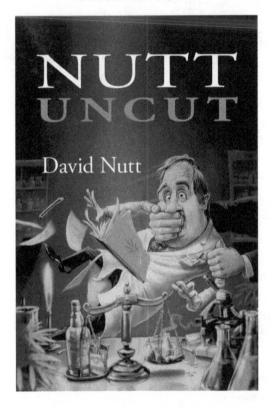

A direct challenge to politicians and others by a world expert on drugs. David Nutt regularly hit the headlines as the UK's forthright Drugs Czar (Chair of the Advisory Council on the Misuse of Drugs), not least when fired by the Home Secretary in 2009 for his 'inconvenient' views. In *Nutt Uncut* he explains how he survived ill-judged political and media vilification to establish the respected charity Drug Science, with the aim of telling the truth about drugs.

Paperback | ISBN 978-1-909976-85-6 | 2021 | 256 pages

www.WatersidePress.co.uk

CPSIA information can be obtained
at www.ICGtesting.com
Printed in the USA
LVHW030001251121
704328LV00008B/946